Intermittent Fasting
for Women Over 50

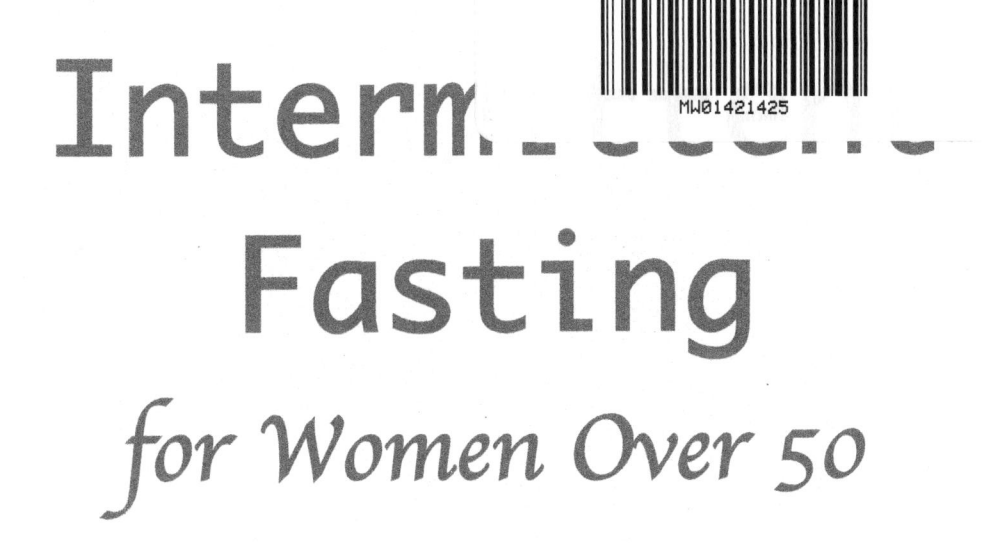

A Guide to Intermittent Fasting and Increased Metabolism and Energy Levels. A Healthy Alternative to Detoxify the Body and Rejuvenate!

By

Emma Sanchez

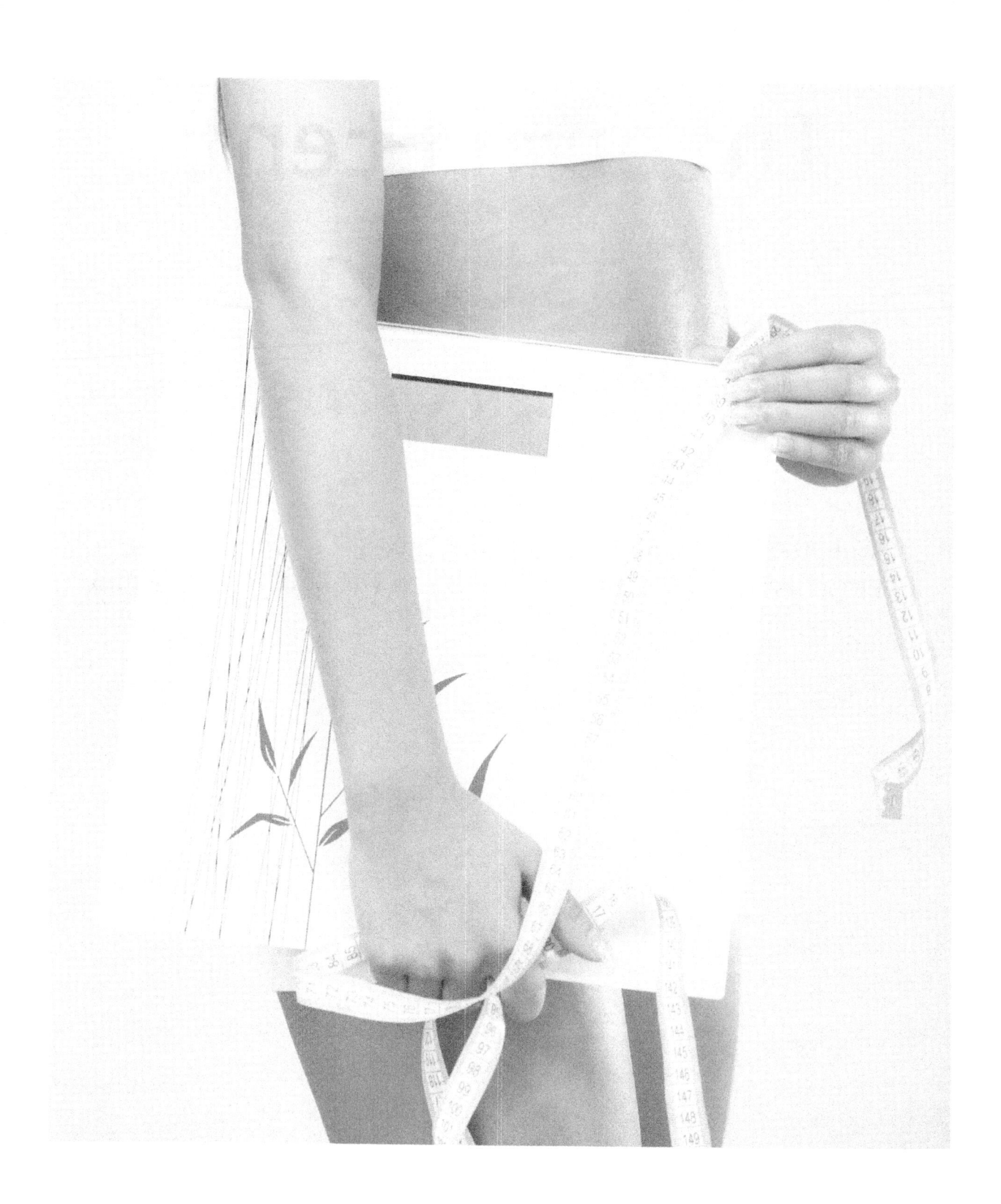

© **Copyright 2022 by Emma Sanchez - All rights reserved**.

This document is geared towards providing exact and reliable information in regard to the topic and issue covered.

- From a Declaration of Principles which was accepted and approved equally by a Committee of the American Bar Association and a Committee of Publishers and Associations.

In no way is it legal to reproduce, duplicate, or transmit any part of this document in either electronic means or printed format. All rights reserved.

The information provided herein is stated to be truthful and consistent, in that any liability, in terms of inattention or otherwise, by any usage or abuse of any policies, processes, or directions contained within is the solitary and utter responsibility of the recipient reader. Under no circumstances will any legal responsibility or blame be held against the publisher for any reparation, damages, or monetary loss due to the information herein, either directly or indirectly.

Respective authors own all copyrights not held by the publisher.

The information herein is solely offered for informational purposes and is universal, and the presentation of the information is without a contract or any guaranteed assurance.

The trademarks that are used are without any consent, and the publication of the trademark is without permission or backing by the trademark owner. All trademarks and brands within this book are for clarifying purposes only and are owned by themselves, not affiliated with this document.

contents

INTRODUCTION 9
CHAPTER 1: WHAT IS INTERMITTENT FASTING? 11
   SCIENCE AND INTERMITTENT FASTING 12
   LONGEVITY AND INTERMITTENT FASTING 13
   HOW DOES IT WORK? 13
   EFFECTS ON HORMONES AND CELLS 14
   INTERMITTENT FASTING DRAWBACKS 15
   RISKS FOR INTERMITTENT FASTING 16

CHAPTER 2: TYPES OF INTERMITTENT FASTING 17
   FASTING 19
   TIME-RESTRICTED FASTING 19
   OVERNIGHT FASTING 20
   EAT STOP EAT 21
   WHOLE-DAY FASTING 21
   ALTERNATE-DAY FASTING 22
   CHOOSE-YOUR-DAY FASTING 22

CHAPTER 3: STAYING MOTIVATED DURING INTERMITTENT FASTING .. 24
   INTERMITTENT FASTING 26
   MAKE IT A NEW NORMAL PRACTICE 26
   BE STRATEGIC 27
   FIND WAYS TO MOTIVATE YOURSELF 27
   DON'T STOP TRYING NEW THINGS 27
   KEEP IN MIND YOUR GENUINE REQUIREMENTS 27
   DRINK PLENTY OF WATER 28
   CALORIE CONSUMPTION 28
   ALTERNATIVE ACTIVITIES 29

CHAPTER 4: HOW MUCH WEIGHT CAN BE LOST WITH INTERMITTENT FASTING? 30
   LOSE WEIGHT IN A HEALTHY AND USEFUL MANNER BY FASTING 31
   WHAT TO EAT WHEN INTERMITTENT FASTING REGARDING WEIGHT REDUCTION? 33
   WHAT'S THE DIFFERENCE BETWEEN SHEDDING POUNDS AND TRIMMING DOWN ON FAT? 34
   WHY IT IS POSSIBLE THAT YOU WON'T SEE RESULTS? 34

CHAPTER 5: PSYCHOLOGICAL EFFECTS OF INTERMITTENT FASTING ... 36
   INFLUENCE OF FOOD 37
   OPTIMIZING EATING TIMES 38
   MOOD SWINGS 39

    Risk of Eating Disorder 40
    Impact on Cognitive Thinking 41

CHAPTER 6: STRESS-FREE RECIPES EATING PLAN 43
    Get Rid Of Tension In The Kitchen 44
    Organize Your Kitchen 44
    Prepare A Strategy And A Plot 45
    Be A Wise Cook 46
    Advice From The Experts 48
    Make Use Of A Service That Delivers Recipe Boxes 49

CHAPTER 7: HIDDEN POWER OF INTERMITTENT FASTING TO CONTROL MOOD, ANXIETY, AND DEPRESSION 50
    Can Intermittent Fasting Boost Mood? 52
    How Food Impacts Mood? 53
    Why Does Fasting Affect Brain Health And Mood? 54
    Mental Function 54
    Optimized Eating 54

CHAPTER 8: HEALTHY EATING TIPS AND TRICKS 56
    Varying Nutritional Requirements Of Women 57
    Diet Tips for PSM Symptoms 59
    Dietary recommendations during pregnancy 60

CHAPTER 9: EXERCISE COMBINED WITH FASTING 62
    Insulin Sensitivity 63
    Testosterone Levels Rise 64
    Oxidation of Fat That Is More Efficient 64
    The Numerous Advantages of Engaging in Physical Activity while Fasting 64
    Why Going Out During Intermittent Fasting Might Not Be Effective 65
    When Should You Next Have a Meal? 66

CHAPTER 10: BREAKFAST RECIPES 67
    Keto Turmeric Milkshake 68
    Spinach Frittata 68
    Fat-Burning Coconut Cookies 69
    Baked Perfect Potato 69
    Savory Oats and Roasted Veggies Bowl 70
    Farro Chicken Bowls 70
    Pumpkin-Peanut Butter Single-Serve Muffins 71
    Breakfast Sausage Casserole 72
    Crustless Broccoli Cheese Quiche 72
    Fruits Breakfast Salad 73
    Pesto Egg Casserole 73
    Kiwi Shake 73

- GREEK TOAST 73
- MUSHROOMS BITES 74
- WHOLE-GRAIN PANCAKES 74
- OMELET WITH ASPARAGUS 74
- BREAKFAST GRANOLA 74
- BREAKFAST EGG TOASTS 75
- RICOTTA TOAST WITH PISTACHIOS AND HONEY 75
- GRANNY SMITH APPLES 75
- SPICED CONGEE WITH DATES 76
- HAM AND CHEDDAR OMELETS 76
- BASIC OATMEAL 76
- CHORIZO, TOMATO & GRILL CHILI FRITTATA 76
- MUESLI WITH COCONUT, OATS & BANANAS 77
- STEEL-CUT OATS 77

CHAPTER 11: LUNCH RECIPES **78**

- PEPPER AND PESTO CHICKEN PANINI 79
- CAPRESE SANDWICH 79
- FETA QUICHE 79
- ASIAN MEATBALL 80
- AVOCADO AND GRILLED CHICKEN 80
- FETTUCCINE ALFREDO PASTA 81
- CHEESESTEAK SANDWICH 81
- MEATBALL SOUP 82
- MASHED CAULIFLOWER 82
- BUM'S LUNCH 83
- HIGH-TEMP PORK ROAST 83
- CHICKPEA SALAD WITH TOMATO AND RED ONION 84
- CHICKEN & BACON CAESAR SALAD 84
- BARBECUED POUSSINS WITH CHILI CORN SALSA 84
- KALE LASAGNA WITH MEAT SAUCE 85
- BLUE CHEESE, SPINACH MEAT LOAF MUFFINS 86
- SYRIAN RICE WITH MEAT 86
- DEER MEAT 86
- SICILIAN MEAT ROLL 87
- CHICKEN-APRICOT CASSEROLE 87
- PASTA WITH GRILLED CHICKEN, WHITE BEANS, AND MUSHROOMS 88
- LEMON ROSEMARY CHICKEN 88
- CHICKEN ZUCCHINI PIE 89
- CHICKEN ETOUFFEE 89
- TASTY FISH FILLETS 89
- GRILLED DORY FISH 90
- TUNA AND BROCCOLI PASTA 90
- CHICKEN WITH HERBS 91

CHAPTER 12: DINNER RECIPE 92

- Sweetened Potato Curry with Chickpeas 93
- Black Eyed Crock Pot Peas 93
- Chicken Sheet Pan Brussel Sprouts 94
- Cauliflower Thin Crust Pizza 94
- Baked Potato Dish 95
- Black Bean Burrito 95
- Super Tilapia Parmesan 96
- Pineapple and Ham Dinner 96
- Savory Oatmeal with Mushrooms 97
- Spice-Rubbed Ribs 97
- Chinese Pork Ribs 97
- Popcorn Shrimp 98
- Lemon Rosemary Salmon 98
- Bowl Of Avocado And Tahini Paste 99
- Cajun-spiced Tilapia 99
- Tuna Melts 99
- Grilled Cod 100
- Cod and Green Bean Curry 100
- Calamari Salad 100
- Acorn Squash with Stuffing 101
- Mussels Steamed in Coconut Broth 101
- Caramelized Onions 101
- Italian Style Stuffed Tomatoes 102
- Greek Green Beans & Tomatoes 102
- Orange Flavored Carrots 102
- Basic Lima Beans 102
- Egg and Salsa 103

CHAPTER 13: DESSERT RECIPE 104

- Banana Ice-Cream 105
- Cottage Cheese and Fruit Snacks 105
- Protein Bars 105
- Raspberry Jelly 105
- Cheesecake 106
- Beans Brownies 106
- Avocado Mousse 106
- Fruit Kebabs 107
- Vanilla Soufflé 107
- Strawberries in Dark Chocolate 107
- White bean dip 108
- Hummus with ground lamb 108
- Eggplant dip 108
- Veggie fritters 108

- Bulgur lamb meatballs 109
- Baked apricot dessert 109
- Blackberry chocolate dessert cake 109
- Layered mascarpone & strawberry dessert 110
- Spiced apple dessert 111
- Apple crumble dessert cake 111

CHAPTER 14 -21 DAYS MEAL PLAN 113
CONCLUSION 115

Introduction

You've probably heard the phrase "intermittent fasting" before. Despite its intimidating sounding name, this method is straightforward to carry out. Additionally, it was selected by the public as the most effective weight reduction method for the year 2019. If you are already used to going without food for extended periods, intermittent Fasting won't present any additional challenges. It is also not needed/necessary to have prior knowledge about fasting to engage in the practice of intermittent Fasting; all that is needed is a willingness to do so. Fasting for shorter periods at regular intervals has gained widespread popularity and is now routine for many people. It has many more benefits to offer than you may think at first glance. This great time of age above 50 in a woman's life is the golden decade. They fully accept themselves and make every effort to have a happy and serene existence. What a lovely world it would be if things were always like that. Unfortunately, this is not the case, and even while women may live a wonderful life beyond the age of 60, several issues may prevent them from continuing their lifestyle. The female body goes through a natural process of transformation as it ages.

If a woman has a higher proportion of lean muscle to fat, her metabolism will be higher. By changing their lifestyles, women could affect the pace at which they age. Intermittent Fasting is one of the things that may be done to slow down the aging process that naturally occurs in the body (IF). In recent years, intermittent Fasting has garnered a growing amount of interest due to the many health advantages and the fact that it does not restrict the kind of foods that may be consumed throughout the fasting periods. The benefits of intermittent Fasting include enhancements to metabolic function and mental health and the potential for cancer prevention in certain cases.

Additionally, it may assist ladies over 60 in awarding against certain nerve, muscle, and joint ailments. It is not a diet(regimen) so much as a style of life that one chooses to live. This diet will aid you in consuming fewer calories daily and provide you with assistance as you continue your path to losing weight. Some women who practice IF choose to do alternate-day Fasting, in which they normally eat on alternate days and consume just 25 percent of their typical daily calorie intake on the days on which they do not fast.

You don't have to exclude whole food groups or restrict your calorie intake to lose weight; rather, it's more of a "lifestyle" than an all-consuming one! Humans have practiced fasting for millennia. When humans lived in hunter-gatherer communities without access to modern comforts like supermarkets and freezers, it was common to experience periods of plenty and shortage. Intermittent Fasting fosters a healthy attitude in addition to physical advantages. It increases brain chemicals that aid in forming new brain cells, preventing Alzheimer's disease, and promoting mental clarity in women. Intermittent Fasting is an excellent technique for a lady in her 50s to feel more confident than she was in the past.

Chapter 1: What is Intermittent Fasting?

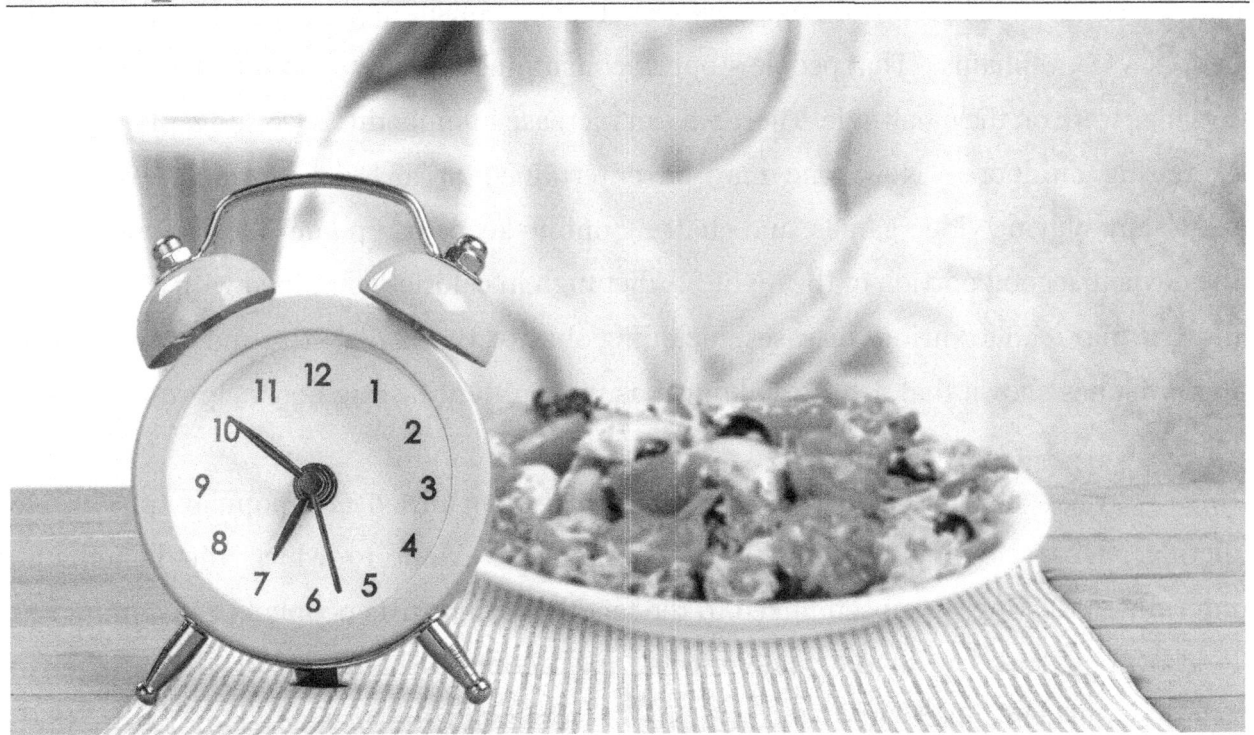

In the period-restricted eating pattern known as intermittent fasting, participants normally eat for the first eight hours before forgoing food consumption for the remaining 16 hours of the day. It is ideal for arranging one's daily meals to get the most out of their nutritional potential. It is more beneficial to give your body more time to absorb meals than to reduce the number of calories you consume. The primary focus of this eating plan is on shifting the timing of your meals rather than changing the foods you eat.

The amount of time spent eating is limited during an intermittent fast. It's possible that eating just one meal per day or fasting for a certain amount of time will help the body burn more fat. Additionally, there can be some positive effects on one's health. Mark Mattson, a neurologist at Johns Hopkins, has spent the better part of the last quarter-century researching it. He asserts that human bodies have been created to endure without sustenance for a period that might range from hours to days to weeks. People who lived before agriculture were hunter-gatherers and had to be able to survive and even thrive for extended periods without access to food. Had to: The pursuit of wild game and collecting nuts and berries requires a significant investment of time and effort. It is now much leisurely/easier to maintain a healthy weight than fifty years ago. "There are no computers, and TV shows finished at midnight; people stopped consuming because people went to bed," says C. Williams. "That people stopped consuming because people went to bed." The servings were on the small side. There was an increase in individuals working, playing, and exercising outdoors. "Now, one may be entertained at any day or night. Watching television, playing video games, and chatting online keeps us up late. We eat throughout the day and a good portion of the night." A diet high in calories combined with a sedentary lifestyle may lead to various diseases, including obesity, type 2 diabetes, and heart disease. Research has shown that a strategy known as intermittent fasting may help reverse these habits.

In recent years, alternating periods of eating with fasting have been a popular approach to dieting. "Our scientific community is split on the extent to which the benefits of intermittent fasting have been linked to the fact that this assists people in consuming less food overall. If you want the same effects, how about cutting down on the number of calories you consume?" At the University of Alabama, Ph.D. candidate Courtney M. Peterson is researching time-restricted eating, a kind of intermittent fasting.

The diet that is greatest for your health is that you can stick to while still having the most fun in life. Help may be found via medical professionals and ongoing research. According to Dr. Peterson, it is difficult to maintain a completely devoid of calories fast. "People remain with them momentarily, but they become hungry," she said. "People stay with them temporarily." It is possible to say that this kind of fasting is the easiest to follow. A longer period spent fasting each night allows you to burn off some of your stored glycogen. It accomplishes a pair of goals. It makes it possible for the body to burn fat slower. According to Dr. Peterson, it may also help the body get rid of extra salt, which will result in a decrease in your blood pressure.

Science and Intermittent Fasting

There is also an element of science involved, namely, creating HGH in your body. But earlier/before I go into it, let me first explain why. Our bodies produce insulin on their own to store glycogen from carbohydrates. We are people that eat three square meals a day, and many of the foods we eat are high in both sugar and fat. As a direct consequence of this, we continue to pack on the pounds. Gaining weight is a direct result of consuming a diet rich in glucose. This process is reversed by intermittent fasting, making it possible for our cells to utilize glucose stored in our bodies. The breakdown of cells, known as catabolism, is responsible for weight loss. HGH is produced because of the demand for glucose placed on the body. Therefore, consuming food regularly inhibits the production of HGH. HGH is wonderful for muscle regeneration and burning fat and its ability to regulate metabolism. HGH production may be raised by as much as five times using intermittent fasting.

Longevity and Intermittent Fasting

There is also a scientific component: creating HGH inside your body. But first, allow me to explain the reason why. Insulin is produced naturally inside our bodies for glycogen stored from carbohydrates. In the society in which we now reside, most meals are eaten at regular intervals, and most foods are high in both sugar and fat content. Because of this, our weight continues to creep up on us steadily. Gaining weight is one of the side effects of consuming a diet rich in glucose. This process is turned around by intermittent fasting, enabling our cells to utilize glucose stored in our bodies. The breakdown of cells or catabolism causes weight loss. HGH is produced because of the necessity that the body has for glucose. Therefore, eating often inhibits the production of HGH. HGH helps regulate metabolism and has positive effects on muscle regeneration and the burning of fat. Intermittent fasting may enhance the body's HGH production by five times.

How Does it Work?

Eating normally but going without food for certain periods at regular intervals is intermittent fasting. Try restricting you're eating to only eight hours a day and going without food for the remaining 16 hours. Alternately, you might have only one meal each day, two times per week. There are a few different approaches to intermittent fasting. Mattson notes that when the body runs out of sugar, it will start burning fat for fuel. He refers to this process as metabolic switching. According to Mattson, "intermittent fasting is not common among Americans since most people eat continually throughout the day." If a person consumes three meals and three snacks daily but does not engage in physical activity, that person is functioning on empty calories and is not, as a result, burning fat. The benefits of intermittent fasting come from lengthening the amount of time that passes between meals, during which your body continues to burn calories and fat.

Drinking just water and calorie-free liquids between meals is OK, including black tea and coffee. In addition, "eating normally" is not synonymous with "getting mad." If you pack your meals with high-calorie, unhealthy items such as fried foods and desserts, you won't be able to reduce weight or improve your health. Williams appreciates the flexibility of intermittent fasting, which enables him to eat and enjoy a wider range of foods. She notes that the organization promotes "encouraging individuals to enjoy eating nutritious cuisine." According to her, having a pleasant time while eating together is enjoyable and beneficial to overall health. Along with most dietitians, Williams thinks that the Mediterranean diet is an outstanding example of how one should eat, regardless of whether one practices intermittent fasting. Whole grains, green leafy vegetables, healthy fats, and lean proteins are four food groups that will never steer you wrong.

In the end, the whole shebang comes down to individual preference. "Be ready to explore," recommends Taylor to anybody interested in giving intermittent fasting a try. "There is a possibility of learning via trial and error." However, according to Taylor, some people have difficulty and need to reduce their time spent fasting.

Effects on Hormones and Cells

Your body goes through cellular and molecular reorganization whenever you fast. It alters hormone levels and makes the fat that has been accumulated easier to reach. In addition to this, your cells may adjust gene expression and repair damage. When you fast, your body goes through a lot of changes, including the following:

Human growth hormone (HGH): Its levels increase by five. It is beneficial to both the decrease of fat and muscle growth.

Insulin: Sensitivity improves as insulin levels drop significantly. When insulin levels are low, access to body fat is made easier.

Cell repair: When you fast, your cells can heal themselves. Autophagy is involved in which cells disassemble and dispose of damaged or outdated proteins.

Gene expression: Certain modifications influence both longevity and disease resistance. The hormonal changes, cellular function, and gene expression improvements that result from intermittent fasting are the source of the health benefits of this eating pattern.

Intermittent fasting Drawbacks

When IF doesn't work out as planned, it's usually since the artificial time limit doesn't truly influence something that would move their aims ahead. Intermittent fasting may be a nuisance or a hindrance for people, regardless of whether they are trying to improve their athletic ability or weight reduction.

When it comes to weight reduction, we may witness an unsuccessful cycle

- Their body does not respond well to a fast lasting for sixteen hours.
- They are hungry and consume excessive food throughout the allotted eating window of eight hours.

They don't lose weight since they consume enough food during the 8-hour timeframe to compensate for the 16-hour fast earlier in the day. The fast imposed an artificial time limit on them, but it did not change their overall objectives.

When it comes to athletic performance, the 16-hour fast might lead to two different issues

- Makes it difficult to consume enough protein.
- It becomes more difficult to get the fuel necessary for an energetic day.

Protein is often a consideration for anybody working to improve their strength. If it is more difficult for you to satisfy your protein requirements within an eight-hour meal window, you are creating it more challenging for yourself to meet your achievement nutritional requirements.

Or, if you are participating in an activity that demands stamina, such as going for a walk, mountain biking, rock climbing, or taking an extended lesson in martial arts, skipping breakfast is often not a decent/good idea since it will negatively impact your performance. The 16:8 cycle generates two food-related issues

- Even if hungry, you fast for 16 hours.
- Even if full, you eat more throughout the 8-hour interval.
- Because you suppress hunger and fullness signals, you lose touch with them.
- You obey an unreasonable rule.

Four signs why 16:8 fasting isn't good for you

- The 16-hour fast is unhealthy.
- The 8-hour eating window hurts.
- It makes automated food intake tougher.
- Your food connection is deteriorating.

Risks for Intermittent Fasting

It is essential/important to note that intermittent fasting is not appropriate for everyone, particularly pregnant women, children, diabetics, and those with other chronic diseases. According to the advice of Taylor, an individual who is at risk for merely an eating issue should not engage in any fasting diet. Because of its restrictions, intermittent fasting puts some individuals at a greater risk of engaging in binge eating. If someone wishes to participate in intermittent fasting, they need to be aware of its risks. It's been related to impatience, weariness, temperature sensitivity, a never-ending hunger, and poor outcomes at work and in activities. Finally, make an appointment with your primary care physician to discuss your options. They are the most qualified to provide advice to anybody about whether the many different intermittent fasting methods are beneficial for a particular individual.

Chapter 2: Types of Intermittent Fasting

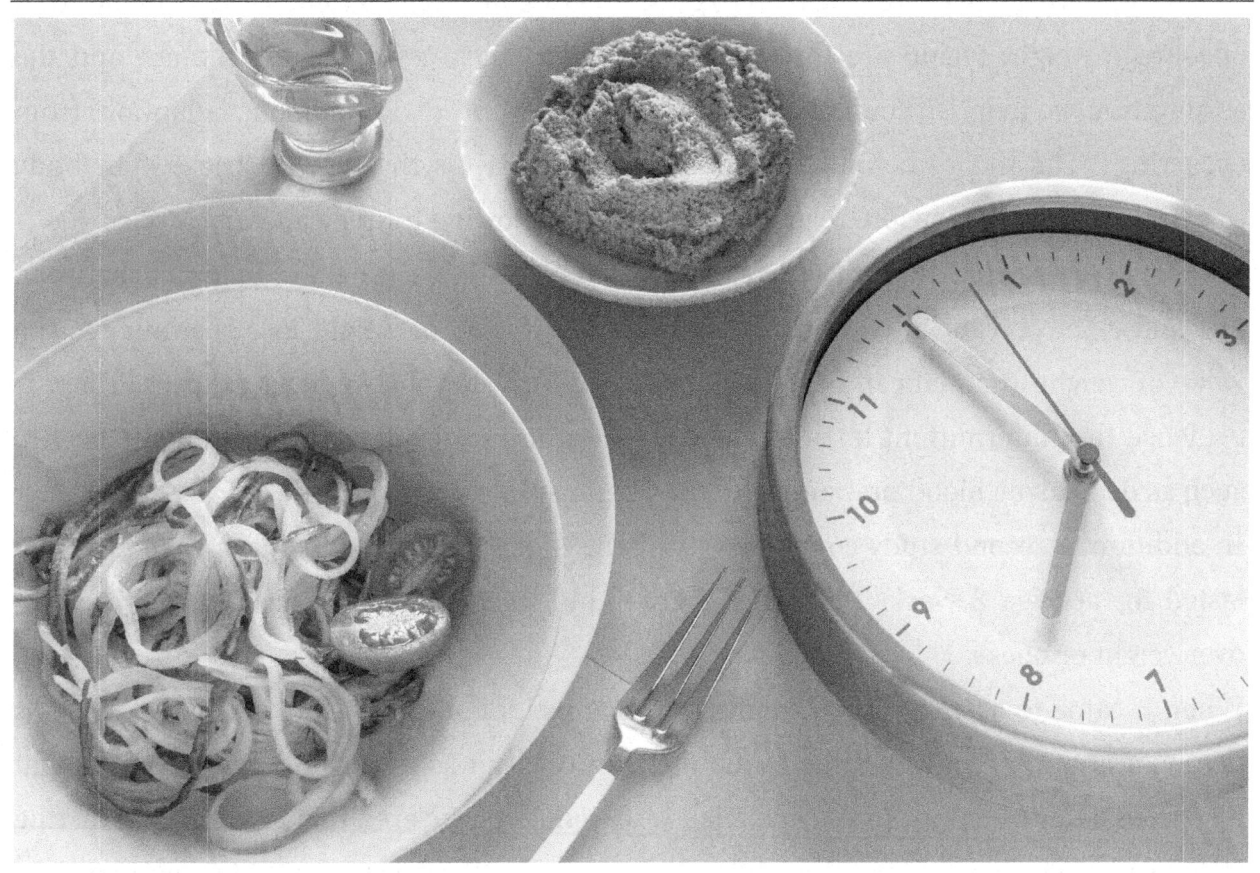

There are two schools of thinking that explain why intermittent fasting (IF) an effective strategy for weight reduction may be. The first is that "Periods of fasting cause net fewer calories, thus you lose weight," as explained by Rekha Kumar, MD, endocrinology, diabetic, and metabolism expert who works just at Comprehensive Weight Command Center at Weill Metropolitan Medicine in New York.

You may be familiar with the well-known research project The Biggest Loser. After six years, the researchers did a follow-up with the people who had participated in the TV show. They found that despite their preliminary impressive losing weight, the participants had gained the majority of the weight back, and their metabolic activity had slowed to the point where they burned a significantly lower number of calories than was expected.

Although further study is required to determine the safety and efficacy of intermittent fasting (IF), one of the purported advantages of this method is that it may avoid the sputtering of the metabolism. According to Kumar, "most individuals who attempt to lose weight by dieting and exercising tend to go off the wagon and gain weight." "Hormones that encourage weight regain are thrown into full gear, such as hunger hormones, and the assumption is that IF could be a method to prevent that metabolic adaption from occurring." The theory behind intermittent fasting (IF) is that it will "trick" your body towards losing weight before reaching a plateau by allowing for typical eating cycles.

According to research, intermittent fasting (IF) may result in a weight reduction of between one and eight percent of one's starting weight. This level of weight loss is similar to the value of weight loss that can be anticipated when on a diet that reduces calories. There is evidence that intermittent fasting may enhance other aspects of cardiometabolic health, such as decreasing blood pressure and lowering insulin resistance.

In addition, a second study conducted its analysis of 11 IF clinical studies, each of which lasted for at least 8 weeks (about 2 months) and included individuals who were either overweight or obese.

When it came to assisting participants in losing weight and body fat, nine of those trials demonstrated that an IF regimen was just as successful as a conventional diet (one that restricted calories daily). In the last trial, researchers discovered that intermittent fasting (IF) for 12 weeks (about 3 months) did not impact cholesterol levels but did result in weight loss and a reduction in systolic blood pressure.

It is essential to remember that researching the human lifespan entails more complexity than only focusing on weight reduction. Because of this, the majority of the studies that seem to indicate that IF contributes to a longer life have been conducted in animals, notably fruit flies.

Another study has shown that the metabolic benefit of IF is that it changes your body into ketosis of ketosis, which is the technical process in the keto diet. Ketosis is when your body burns fat for fuel rather than carbs, and it is one of the benefits of the keto diet.

In addition to their benefits on weight reduction, experts believe that ketones may also activate the body's natural repair mechanisms, which might, in the long run, provide protection against illness and the ravages of aging.

However, it is essential to ensure that your expectations about IF are realistic. Because so much research has been conducted on animals, it is challenging to extrapolate those findings to humans, who are certainly capable of independent thought and must contend with the impacts of lifestyle issues such as stress at work, crazy schedules, comfort eating, and cravings, to name a few. These factors can impact an individual's adherence to a particular diet. Although intermittent fasting (IF) shows promise, it is not significantly more successful than every diet.

The fact that IF may be executed in such a wide variety of methods is a positive development. Suppose you are interested in carrying this out. In that case, you may choose the strategy that will mesh most naturally with your way of life, significantly improving your chances of success. Here are seven:

Fasting

One of the most used IF approaches is to use this procedure. The plan is to eat regularly for five days (don't monitor calories), and then on the sixth and seventh days, consume either 500 or 600 calories (about 48 minutes of running) per day, depending on whether you are a woman or a man. The days of the fast are days that you choose for yourself.

If you become hungry when you are on a fasting week, all you have to do is think forward to the following day, when you will be able to "feast" once again. It is the theory behind intermittent fasting, in which you go for brief periods without eating. Instead of reducing their caloric intake for the whole week, these individuals could find more success with the 5:2 method.

However, if you plan on performing a lot of intense exercise on a given day, it is not a good idea to go without food at that time. Consider whether or not this kind of fasting will be compatible with your training regimen if you are currently preparing for cycling or running competition (or if you are running high-mileage weeks). You might also see a dietitian who specializes in athletics.

Time-Restricted Fasting

During this kind of intermittent fasting (IF), you select an eating window daily, which should leave you with a time of fasting that lasts anywhere from 14 to 16 hours. Shemek suggests that women eat for no or more than 14 hours a day to avoid adverse effects on their hormones. According to Shemek, "Fasting encourages autophagy, the natural 'cellular housekeeping' process where the stomach clears debris and other things which come in the way of a health of mitochondria." This process starts when the liver glycogen stores are depleted and continues when the body is fasting. According to her, carrying out these steps may assist enhance the metabolism of fat cells and improving insulin activity.

For example, suppose you follow this strategy. In that case, you can decide to limit your meals to 9 am to 5 pm. According to Kumar, this strategy may work particularly well for someone who already eats supper at an early hour and has a family. If this is the case, then a sizable portion of fasting time is spent sleeping. Depending on that, when you set up your window, you also do not technically have to "miss" any meals while you are doing this. However, this will be contingent on your ability to maintain consistency. Daily periods of fasting may not be the best choice for you if you have an unpredictable schedule or if you want or need the flexibility to do things like go out for a late- on the town with a date, go to happy hour, or go out for breakfast on occasion.

Overnight Fasting

This method, which is the easiest, requires abstaining from food for twelve consecutive hours daily. Take, for instance, the scenario in which you decide to finish your meal at 7 pm, call it quits for the day, and then start eating again at 7 am the following morning with breakfast. At the 12-hour point, autophagy will still occur, but the advantages to cells will be far less significant, according to Shemek. It is the bare minimum amount of time she suggests being without food.

The simplicity of this approach is one of the method's many advantages. Also, you don't need to skip meals; all you're doing is getting rid of a bedtime appetizer if you were eating one to initiate with if that's the only change you make. However, this technique does not make the most of the benefits of fasting. If you are trying to lose weight by fasting, having a shorter fasting window will allow more time to feed, and it is unlikely that this will help you cut down on the number of calories you take in.

Eat Stop Eat

Author Brad Pilon is credited for developing this strategy, detailed in his novel "Eat Stop Eat: The Shocking Truth That Makes It Easy Again to Lose Weight." His emphasis on adaptability sets his method apart from others of its kind. Expressed, he promotes the concept that all involved in fasting are temporarily abstaining from eating food. You commit to a strength exercise regimen and fast for either one or two consecutive periods of 24 hours each week.

Eating responsibly is returning to a regular way of eating, wherein you don't binge eat because you recently fasted, but where you also don't limit yourself with an unhealthy diet or eat more than you need to survive. According to Pilon, the most effective strategy for fat removal is to mix periodic fasting with a regular strength exercise. You permit yourself to consume a little greater total calories on the five or six days of the week when you are not fasting if you subject yourself to one or more 24-hour fasts. It makes it simpler and more pleasurable to finish the year with a calorific deficit while avoiding the impression that one must be on an extremely restrictive diet.

Whole-Day Fasting

At this place, you just eat once each day. Shemek notes that some individuals opt to have supper and then wait to eat till the following day's dinner. In the case of whole-day fasting, both fasting periods are practically 24 hours long, beginning with dinner and continuing through lunch the following day, but in the case of the 5:2 diet, the fasting phase is 36 hours (about 1 and a half days) long. For instance, you may have supper on Sunday, then "fast" on Monday by consuming just 500 or 600 units, and then "break" your fast on Tuesday by eating breakfast.

If you want to lose weight, one of the benefits of fasting for the full day is that it makes it very difficult, if not impossible, to consume an entire day's amount of income in a single meal or snack. One meal may not be enough to provide your body with all of the nutrients it requires to perform at its very best, which is one of the drawbacks of this strategy. Not to add, adhering to this strategy is going to be difficult. By the time supper comes around, you could find that you are quite hungry, which may cause you to make decisions that are not the healthiest and high in calories. Consider this: when you are really hungry, the last thing you want is a serving of broccoli. According to Shemek, a common way for individuals to get over their hunger is to drink excessive coffee, which may negatively impact their ability to sleep. If you don't eat anything throughout the day, you could also have brain fog at various points.

Alternate-Day Fasting

Krista Varady, Ph.D., senior nutritional professor at the University of Illinois in Chicago, is credited with having brought widespread attention to this method. People may choose to fast every day, with a "fast" comprising 25 percent of all the daily calorie requirements and non-fasting days being days they eat normally. It is a strategy that many people use to shed extra pounds. Studies have shown that overweight individuals may benefit greatly from alternate-day fasting by reducing their body mass index, BMI, fat mass, or total cholesterol levels.

On days when you are required to fast, you may be anxious about how hungry you would feel. Previous research conducted and published by Dr. Varady and his colleagues discovered that the negative effects of alternate-day fasting, such as hunger, began to subside by the second week of the diet, and by the fourth week, the participants reported feeling more satisfied while following the diet. The fact that participants in the experiment reported that they never were "full" during the trial duration made it difficult to adhere to this strategy, which was the experiment's primary limitation.

Choose-Your-Day Fasting

This approach to IF is more along the lines of a choose-your-own-adventure book. According to Shemek, you may undertake the time-restricted fasting in which you starve yourself for 16 hours and then eat normally for eight hours once every other day, once or twice a week, etc. That suggests that you may have a typical day of eating on Sunday, in which case you might stop eating at eight o'clock in the evening. After that, you might start eating once more on Monday at midday. In practice, this is equivalent to missing breakfast several times a week.

Something to bear in mind is that the studies on the influence that missing breakfast has on one's ability to lose weight have produced contradictory results. There is little data to support the hypothesis that missing breakfast impacts one's weight. However, some studies have indicated that having breakfast might moderate affect one's ability to shed extra pounds.

Additionally, additional studies have shown a correlation between missing breakfast and an increased risk of death from cardiovascular disease. This strategy is more of a go-with-the-flow approach, which means that you can make things work with a timetable that varies from week to week. It may be easy to adjust to your living and flexible. On the other hand, a more relaxed strategy could only provide modest improvements.

Chapter 3: Staying Motivated during Intermittent Fasting

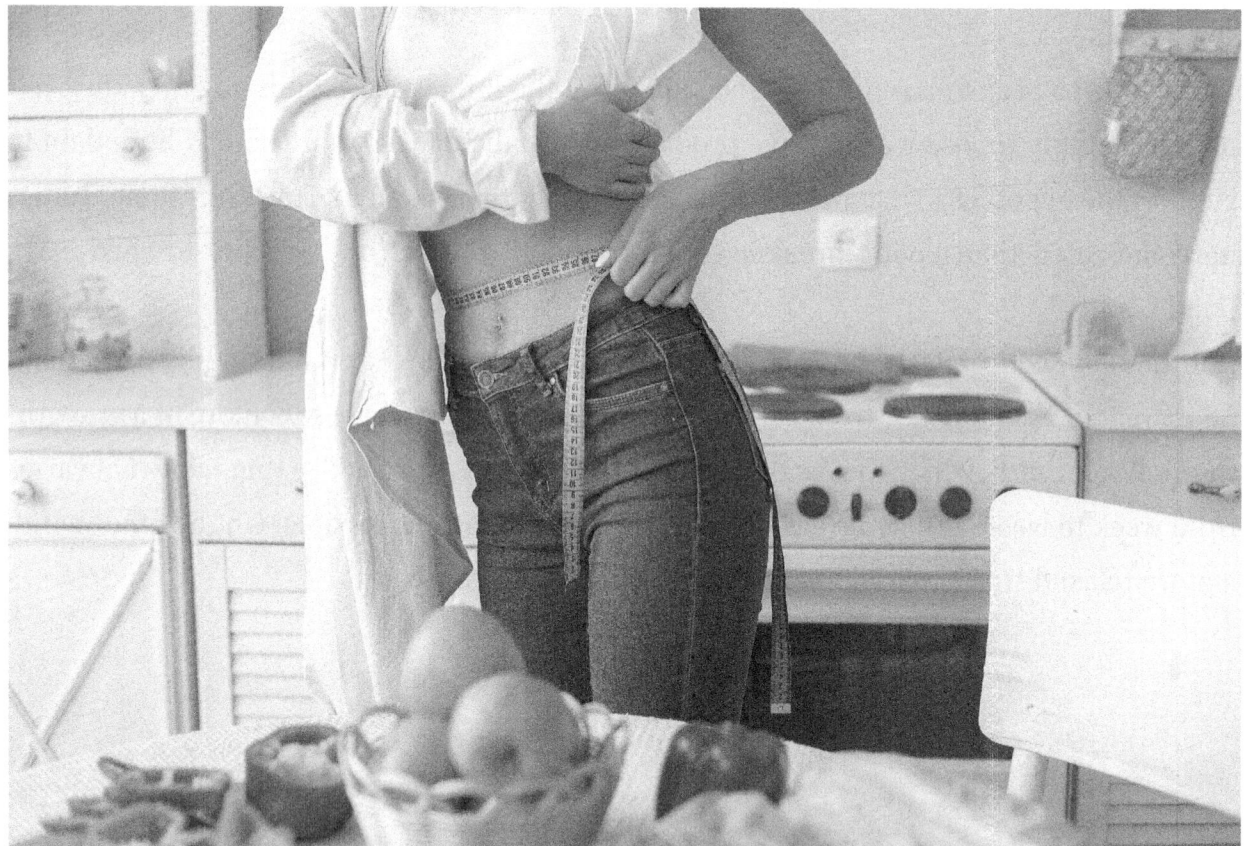

Are you trying to figure out how to maintain your motivation while on a fast? We are completely able to empathize with what you are going through. Fasting on an intermittent basis has seen a recent surge in popularity, particularly among people interested in dieting and fitness. It is an efficient method for shedding extra pounds while maintaining health and physical fitness. Even though it is a straightforward approach to dieting, beginning a new adventure can be nerve-wracking. So, to make the process of intermittent fasting simpler for you, here are some helpful hints. Stay positive and watch your step! When you think of bingeing or quitting, another is written in the palm of your hand, but you don't end up doing either of those things anyhow. And after the day is through, or even when you're in the middle of your fast, you can look down and be surprised to see how many times you haven't given up!

It is of tremendous assistance in fasting, as it is impossible to avoid activities. During a fast, it is helpful to drink a lot of water because it toxins out of your system. Caffein is a stimulating substance that avoiding it may also be helpful. Caffeine is among the "base" nutri that "base" to be balanced out, other foods are required. It is not true at a specific time of day will cause you to experience a state of fasting, so we will not say that it will. We suggest that you consume something at a specific hour on specific days of the week. If you eat something on Monday morning, you will eat something on Friday afternoon, and then you will eat something on Saturday morning if you keep this pattern up. Another helpful hint for consuming your food at a specific time is to skip eating anything from Friday afternoon until Sunday morning and then eat something in the middle of the day. This works out wonderfully, particularly if you have a meeting the first morning. When someone knows they will have an appointment later, they may choose to do this. They will maintain a healthy physical condition because of it. Scientists recommend the practice of intermittent fasting to achieve the greatest outcomes possible. There is no way to acquire what you require in one fell swoop. You run the risk of going overboard, which could lead to you acquiring an unhealthy amount of weight and becoming ill due to the additional eating. We strongly suggest that you create and stick to a plan for each week. You are free to try something new every week. During a test, we believe that no one should ever give up.

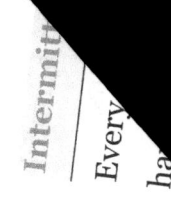

time you experience the sensation that your stomach is about to explode, you should have a small x mark with a red line across it. This is the proposal that we have for you. When doing this, keep in mind the little red x that indicates your stomach will burst if you continue doing this and do not stop right away. That simple x will serve as a powerful incentive for you to initiate a more effective plan to bring your nutrition up to its level to avoid going through that experience again. People like intermittent fasting. It's common for people to have their meals at a specific time of day, and we're positive we won't be forced to contend with that sensation if we don't. If you don't want to deal with it during the week, we advise you to adhere to your primary plan and have everything you always require during the week. A person should also chew their food thoroughly during the week. Take your time, and don't rush. People will typically begin with a light snack and work their way up to a more substantial dinner as the meal progresses. You ought to consider the necessities that your body will call for. You should probably slow down if you have a lot riding on the outcome of your actions. If you have the misfortune of sticking to a plan despite consuming a lot of liquids, you should probably think about joining a support group. On the internet, you can find a plethora of different support groups. It would be to your gain to become a member of one and seek the guidance of people in the community. People can persevere because of the support they receive from their families and friends. If they notice how much you are struggling, they may be able to encourage you to keep going for a little while longer.

Make It a New Normal Practice

Because maximum people are used to eating three times per day, shifting the times we eat can make us feel uneasy. Even if you are not hungry, you will inexplicably get the need to eat anything during lunchtime or breakfast, even if you won't be hungry at those times. Although this may be difficult, consider it the beginning of a new routine. Every new routine requires a period for our body to adjust and become acclimated to it. You must get yourself mentally ready for the kind of change coming. It is going to be challenging at first.

Therefore, it is important that you continually remind yourself why you have decided to follow this diet and remain steadfast in your choice. The process of adopting any new dietary trend is primarily a mental one.

Be Strategic

During the initial days of your intermittent fast, you may find that you wake up every morning feeling extremely hungry. This is quite normal. You may feel an overwhelming want to chew on anything at all. Be aware of what you consume in the hours leading up to the beginning of your fast to avoid putting yourself in a precarious position. Consume an adequate amount of fiber, protein, and whole grains, and above all else, ensure that you drink lots of water. Consuming well-rounded meals rich in satiety before beginning a fast will help you feel satisfied for a longer amount of time.

Find Ways To Motivate Yourself

If you approach it as a challenge, you will find that you can make quick work of it. If you start feeling lethargic, the task will inevitably be challenging. It might be a little simpler if you are thrilled about the notion of fasting; it will make the experience more enjoyable. Convince you that you will have a more positive outlook after completing the task.

Don't Stop Trying New Things

When it comes to intermittent fasting, there is no hard and fast rule; therefore. It is not a given that what is successful for other people will also be successful for you. Although abstaining from food for 18 hours can benefit some people, you should not attempt this if you cannot do so successfully. If you feel that 12 hours is the right amount, stick with it.

Keep In Mind Your Genuine Requirements

Reminding myself that my body needs a specific number of calories each day, no matter what. The hunger you feel outside of that is (usually always) a mix of tension, boredom, and anxiousness and the overpowering societal convention that we're supposed to eat, regardless of our requirements, continually. This causes you to feel hungry. Remind yourselves of that and the truth that hunger is not in and of itself an issue that demands an urgent remedy. Before dinner, we ought to be working on our appetites, which require a couple of hours of hunger that is only moderately intense. Because hunger is a natural aspect of having a human organism, just like the urge to urinate or sleep, we do not need to fight it continuously or silence it. Instead, we should focus on satisfying our needs as best we can. This is not a question of whether you are hungry (within reason).

Drink Plenty of Water

Now is the time to drink a lot of water, and between moisture and herbal tea, you should aim to consume approximately five to six pints of liquid each day. It is not sufficient, but it is unquestionably a significant improvement compared to where we used to be. The combination of caffeine and water helps in the early hours to keep me within this wonderful "fasting" hum where we're super-productive and don't feel hungry, as well as drinking a lot more water throughout the day and while we cooking dinner helps to fill our stomach without necessitating me that you overeat. In addition to the fact that many of the signals that we interpret as hunger are caused by thirst, we, as humans living in a society that is saturated with food marketing, have a really difficult time distinguishing between what is a wholesome amount of food and what is simply eating to please ourselves. It is not a trick to reduce your appetite by drinking more water; rather, it will prevent it from unnecessarily desiring additional fuel.

Calorie Consumption

The question is that most of us don't require that much energy unless we are extremely active, which is why most diets fail when it comes to helping people lose weight. And so, any diet that would keep us below by a sufficient margin requires necessarily — if you are eating 3 meals and a snack — trying to divide those meals up into extremely unsatisfying micro, with no room for error. This is the case for any diet that will keep us below by a sufficient margin. Using calorie requirements as a guide, it would not be difficult for someone to exceed their daily limit with just one purchase of a burger, fries, and a shake. And if you were to split calories into 3 meals and a snack, every one of them would be in the region of 300-400, and a single glass of red wine or spoonful of ice cream would put me over anyway. Additionally, over time, you would gradually acquire weight. It is much simpler for me to eat very little during the day than to have several subpar meals, which can never encompass anything rich but instead delicious, and then be tormented by the worst feeling it is consistent: food guilt. Eating very little throughout the day makes it easier for me to avoid the latter scenario. Nobody should live just like, but if you already must make every meal extremely low in calories to stay within a healthy range, visitors almost certainly will because it is so easy to "mess up." This makes people more depressing to be around than those who go to every meal with feelings of guilt, shame, and rationalization. I've tried many different things, but the only thing that breaks that pattern is IF.

Alternative Activities

The fact that eating out of boredom is a thing ought to go without stating, but it is. It's a thing to eat while doing other things. When you find yourself bored, you should observe something interesting rather than ruminating about food. Some folks get a kick out of viewing only part of an episode of Real Housewives while also playing Threes on their phone and, ideally (eventually), crocheting a scarf. Crucial tasks include finding a few activities that don't require much thought that you can turn to when you find yourself "boredom eating." If you don't, you will find that trying to stuff your face with food is the automatic substitute for what to do if you have lazy parents and a partially occupied brain. People used to puff on cigarettes, but today they mindlessly consume chips. Both are bad for your health, and the solution to both problems is to find something to do with your hands that is more useful (or, at the very least, less directly detrimental).

In conclusion, going through life is about making minor adjustments to your daily patterns. There are times when achieving predetermined objectives is not the most important thing. People who can motivate themselves are more successful than those who cannot. Discover how to maintain your motivation throughout a fast, simply making subtle adjustments to your routine. If you keep acting in that manner, I believe that you will be able to do anything you set your mind to.

Chapter 4: How Much Weight Can Be Lost With Intermittent Fasting?

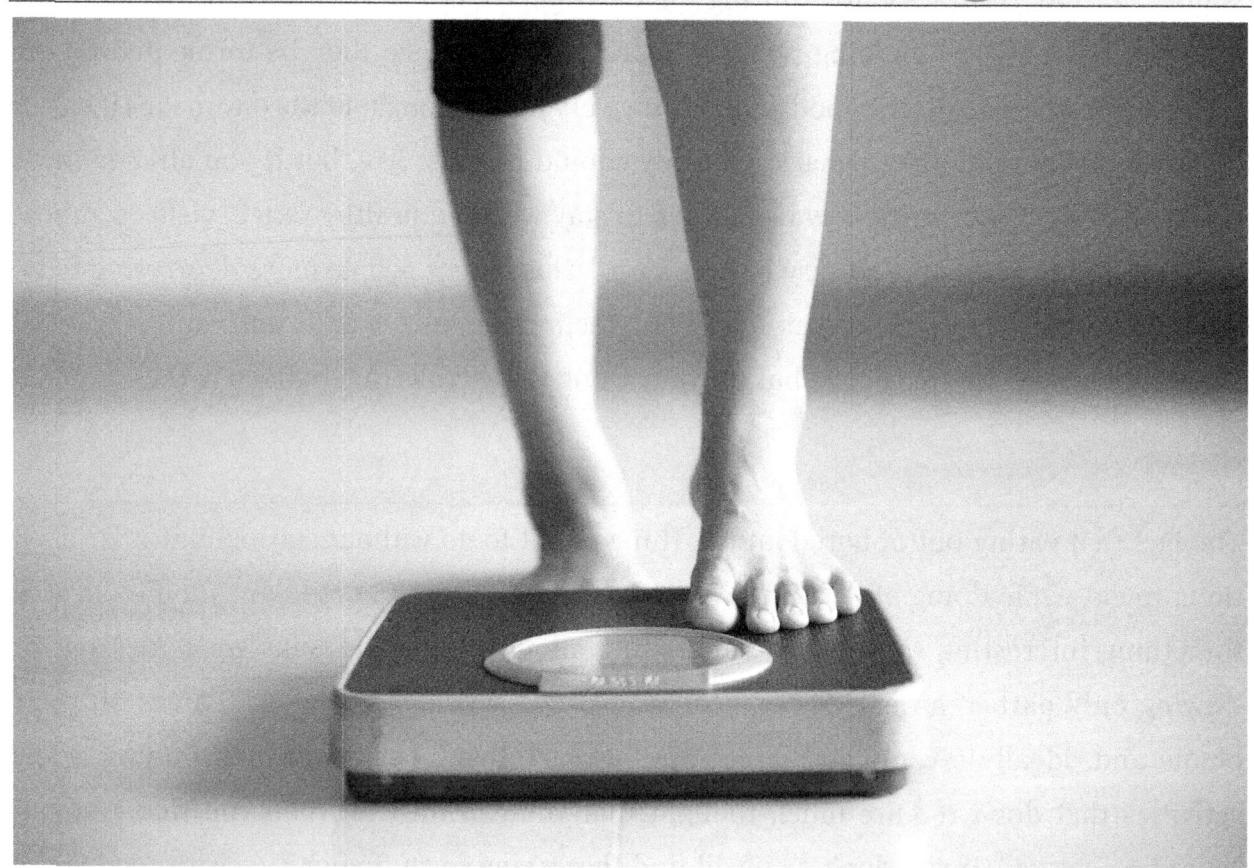

Are you looking to lose weight and are thinking about trying out intermittent fasting? An alternative to continuous fasting is the practice of intermittent fasting. It includes periods of abstinence from food followed by cycles of eating. It entails limiting the amount of time you spend eating each day to a small window of time, between six and eight hours. As the night progresses, our bodies naturally enter a state of fasting that resembles intermittent fasting. You will be fasting if you've been to bed at approximately 10:00 p.m. and don't have breakfast until 7:00 or 8:00 a.m. the following morning. If you can maintain this condition for an additional 6 to 8 hours, you will be able to notice an impact that is far more beneficial. If you finish eating supper by seven o'clock, your next meal won't be until approximately noon the following day. It is the most basic interpretation of what this implies.

The sheer level of dissatisfaction that individuals feel while following conventional diets

drives thousands upon thousands of people every day to seek out risky weight reduction solutions. If you want to get rid of those extra pounds, almost every health website and publication will tell you to cut down on calories. Most of the time, these publications do not give any direction, and some of them encourage diets that are quite restricted and exclude items. Therefore, if you discover that you are stuck in a "yo-yo dieting" cycle, in which you diet, lose weight, regain it, and then diet again, intermittent fasting may be the solution. Weight loss and IF go hand in hand since IF is not your regular diet; hence, weight loss & Intermittent Fasting(IF) go hand in hand. Because intermittent fasting is indeed a lifestyle change, the things you consume and the way you eat them have the potential to assist you in permanently losing those pesky extra pounds.

Intermittent fasting as a strategy for weight reduction is more of an instinctual practice. You will be successful in it as soon as your physical self is prepared to be in harmony with it. In addition to this, it is a natural idea for the human body. It is entirely normal, for instance, for someone who is sick to lose appetite. It happens often. And because our ancestors became hunters & gatherers who did not consume food unless they were successful in bringing down animals or discovering fruits and nuts, our bodies are capable of or well suited to managing IF.

Lose Weight In A Healthy And Useful Manner By Fasting

If someone is obese or overweight, continuing to fast may assist them in losing weight, provided they do it consistently. On the other side, it does not show effectiveness as a diet that restricts calories. Compared to a diet low in calories, a study that lasted for 50 weeks and included 150 obese persons found that fasting two days per week did not result in any substantial weight reduction or improvement in cardiovascular health. However, he should also consider how tough the diet will be. In a study conducted in 2017 on a group of 100 adults who were obese or overweight, those who fasted had a higher dropout rate (38 percent) compared to those who were on a calorie-restricted diet (29 percent) and those who ate normally (27 percent) (26 percent). " Some people have a hard time keeping up with monitoring their food intake on an app consistently. Krista Varady, the principal author of the study and a nutrition specialist at the University of Chicago, suggests that people who have difficulty adhering to daily calorie restrictions could find success with the alternate-day fasting method. We are tricking them into eating less by making them believe that this area is amazing. "In 2017, she made the statement. Certain types of fasting are easier than others, but they also better match the natural circadian cycle of our bodies, therefore lowering insulin levels, increasing hormones that burn fat, and decreasing feelings of hunger. It is possible that eating earlier in the day would be beneficial to us since our metabolism developed to allow for the digestion of food during the day and sleep throughout the night. In the laboratory of Dr. Peterson, 11 people were given food to consume between the hours of 8:00 a.m. & 2:00 p.m. for four days, followed by a control period of 12 hours. The researchers found that restricting meals to a certain amount of time improved the hunger hormone ghrelin levels and increased the amount of fat burned. According to Dr. Peterson's statements, "it has been proven to diminish liver fat," elevated risk for cardiovascular disease and diabetes.

The most common way to lose weight through fasting is called intermittent fasting. By limiting the number of times you eat each day, intermittent fasting makes it possible to cut down on calories. Altering hormone levels is another way that intermittent fasting might assist with weight loss. In addition to this, it promotes an increase in growth hormone while simultaneously lowering insulin levels and elevating norepinephrine levels. Because of hormonal shifts, fasting for shorter periods may cause the body's metabolism to increase by 3.6–14%. By lowering calorie consumption while boosting energy expenditure, intermittent fasting may significantly weight loss. It has been shown that individuals can lose weight by engaging in intermittent fasting. The weight loss of 3–8 percent over 3–24 weeks reported in review research from 2015 is significant compared to most weight loss studies. The average waist circumference of people is reduced by between 4 and 7 percent, which indicates a significant reduction in the amount of harmful belly fat that collects around organs and causes sickness. According to the findings of another study, intermittent fasting is superior to calorie restriction in terms of its ability to prevent muscular atrophy. Keep in mind that the primary reason for its success is that it causes you to consume fewer calories daily. If someone binges and eats excessively during the eating intervals, it is possible that they may not lose weight.

What To Eat When Intermittent Fasting Regarding Weight Reduction?

During the duration of the fast, the only liquid that may be consumed is water. In addition, drinks of any kind, including tea, coffee, and others, are not allowed. Tea, coffee, and other liquids without calories are examples of some additional forms of intermittent fasting.

By lowering insulin levels and minimizing spikes in blood sugar and inflammation, intermittent fasting is an effective method for fat loss. Insulin is the hormone accountable/responsible for storing fat, and by lowering insulin levels, intermittent fasting helps insulin work more effectively. This form of fasting contributes to the body's healing by interrupting the digestive process and rerouting blood flow to sites of the skin that need attention and treatment.

Additionally, BDNF may be stimulated by intermittent fasting. Brain-derived neurotrophic factor, often known as BDNF, is a protein essential for developing new neurons and preserving existing neurons. Because it links one neuron to another, it plays a significant role in the communication process, an essential component of thinking, learning, and the general operation of the brain. Intermittent deprivation of food causes the gene that activates BDNF to become active.

Although a lot of emphases is being paid to the times at then you should be dining, I still want to draw your attention to the importance of eating well-balanced meals, which should include the following components:

- Jowar, raj Gira, bajra, quinoa, oats, and brown rice are complex carbohydrates. Other examples include oats.
- Eggs, poultry, fish, dals, pulses, nuts, and seeds are good, lean protein sources.
- Coconut oil, olive oil, ghee, avocados, nuts, and seeds are examples of foods that contain healthy fats.
- Fruits and vegetables with high fiber content
- Enough water, physical activity, relaxation, and sleep

It is essential to have the understanding that indulging in high-calorie foods such as those that are high in sugar, high fat, refined flour, and highly processed during the eating window would still lead to an inflammatory process and will result in a yo-yo effect in the fat percentage instead of a sustained losing weight effect.

What's the Difference Between Shedding Pounds and Trimming Down on Fat?

It may be thrilling to observe the numbers on the scale decrease as you lose weight. However, the number that appears on the scale does not indicate whether you have shed fat or just general weight. You could believe that the objective of your fitness/health journey is to reduce the amount of body fat you have, but what you want to do is lose weight. The explanation for this is straightforward: when a person reduces their body mass, they might lose any mix of muscle, fluid, fat, and even the size of their organs.

The loss of muscle and fluids is probably not what you want to achieve if your goals are to improve your health and develop muscle so that your body feels & looks more toned. Instead, it would help if you concentrated on reducing your body fat; however, losing over two pounds every week might be detrimental to your efforts.

When you lose more than five pounds in a week, studies, and the recommendations of Doctor Joel Seedman indicate that you will also lose water weight & muscle in addition to your fat weight. Loss of muscle and water may be harmful since it raises the chance of being dehydrated, suffering from vitamin shortages, experiencing a decline in physical and mental function, and increasing the likelihood of putting on the lost weight again. Include strength training in your normal exercise plan so that you may successfully counteract this. Aerobic exercise like running or cycling may help you burn more fat, but resistance training is essential to keep your muscle mass. Additionally, your metabolic rate will increase proportionately with the muscle mass you possess. Standard strength training activities, such as push-ups, squats, and lunges, may help you enhance your body composition by increasing your muscle mass while decreasing your body fat percentage.

Why It is Possible That You Won't See Results?

Even while data shows that intermittent fasting is successful, there are many reasons why you may not get any effects from it. It is possible that you are not consuming enough calories when you are in the fasting window. It may seem counterintuitive. Your body can overcompensate when you significantly limit calories. Your body might undergo metabolic adaptation because of sudden under-consumption. It is a process by which your metabolism becomes more effective at storing fat and utilizing energy, which indicates you will burn fewer calories. Consuming minimally processed, nutrient-dense meals throughout your allotted eating window until you become satisfied is more important than keeping track of your calorie intake and reducing it.

One of the reasons you do not see the results you want maybe that most of the food you consume throughout your meals is highly processed and high in calories. Although there is some evidence that fasting may aid in fat loss, this does not indicate that it is a magic bullet. Keep in mind that you should pile your plate high with complex carbohydrates, lean proteins, and healthy fats.

Finally, throughout your fasting period, you should be sure to consume a lot of water. It is easy to confuse thirst for hunger since dehydration makes you feel fuller and more fulfilled than before. If you are dehydrated while getting close to your eating window, then you may be more likely to pick and consume meals that have been highly processed.

Chapter 5: Psychological Effects Of Intermittent Fasting

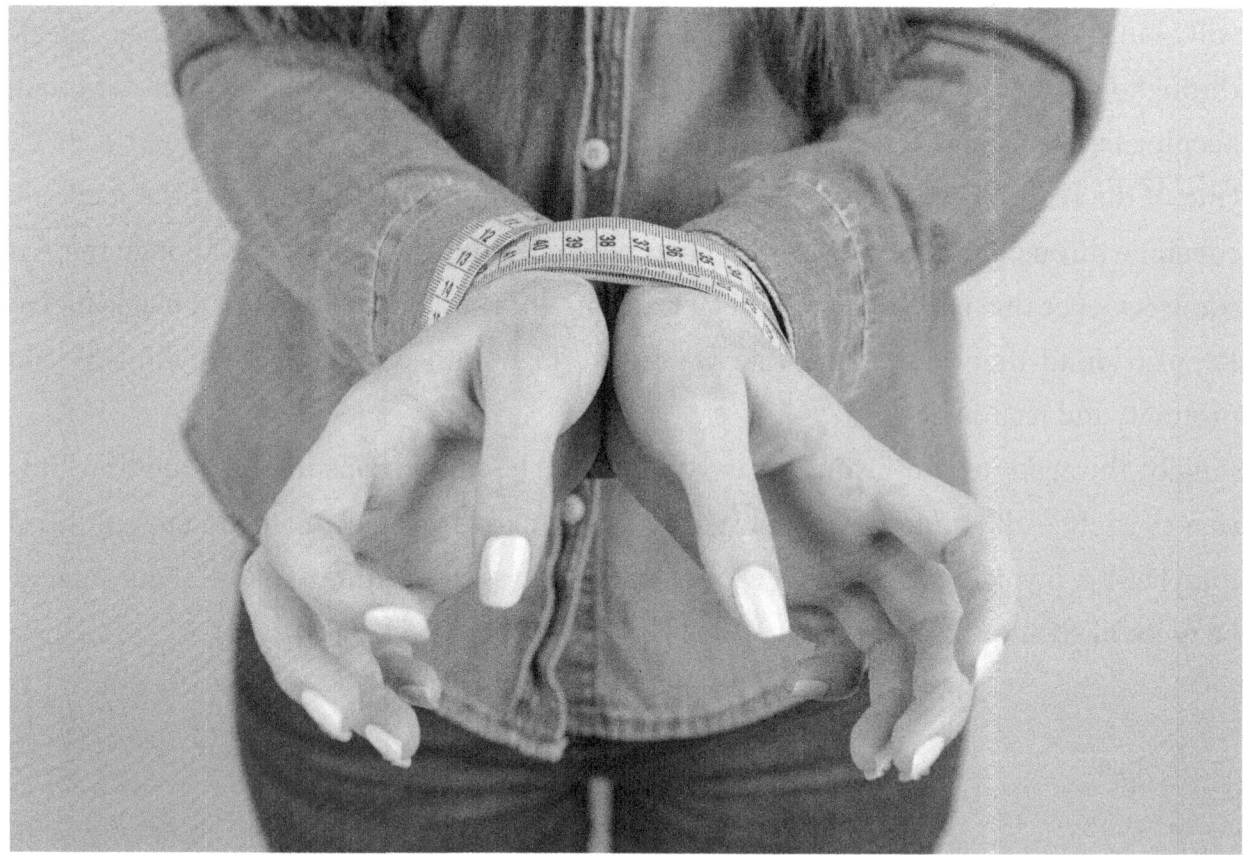

It turns out that the food we eat and the time of day that we eat might affect our brains. Eating is an important element of human existence. It has been demonstrated that irregular eating times may lead to poor psychological health, including sadness and anxiety, cardio-metabolic disorders, and weight gain. It is especially true for adolescents.

It is feasible, and thankfully so, to use the cycles of our meals to reduce bad emotions and promote mental wellness. It all functions as follows: Our internal activities are synchronized at the most efficient periods of the day thanks to the circadian clock, which is triggered by external signals such as the timing of meals and exposure to light. This circuitry has developed in humans to significantly fulfill energy demands that vary day and night. It has resulted in a cyclic pattern to our feeding patterns that match the timetable of the Sun.

Even while the main clock is responsible for regulating metabolic activity throughout the day-night cycle, the rhythms of our meals also affect the main clock. The digestive organs have their internal clocks, and their function demonstrates regular oscillations over a 24-hour cycle. For instance, the ability of the small bowel and liver to digest food, absorb nutrients and burn calories shifts during the day and night.

The capacity of the brain to operate may be negatively impacted whenever the main circadian rhythm in the brain is not coordinated with the cycles of eating. Even though it only makes about two percent of our overall body mass, the brain uses up to percent of our entire body's energy and is especially sensitive to shifts in the number of calories it takes in. It indicates that irregular meal times are certain to have detrimental effects on one's health.

Influence of Food

Even though the underlying processes have not been fully elucidated, there is overlap in the brain circuits responsible for regulating mood and eating. Dopamine is a neurotransmitter that has a significant impact on mood, energy levels, and the experience of pleasure. Additionally, digestive hormones influence dopamine. Patients suffering from depression and bipolar illness have levels of dopamine that are not usual. It is believed that alterations in eating cycles might lead to mental problems.

Inconsistent eating patterns have been hypothesized to contribute to mood disorders and many factors. For instance, people who suffer from depression or bipolar illness often have disrupted internal cycles and inconsistent meal times. Both of these factors contribute considerably to the worsening of mood symptoms. In addition to this, shift workers, who often have erratic eating habits, have been shown to exhibit higher rates of sadness and anxiety in community samples. Despite the evidence to the contrary, monitoring eating cycles is not now a regular component of therapeutic therapy in the majority of psychiatric settings.

Optimizing Eating Times

The question now is, what could be done to make the most of our eating rhythms? Our investigation came across one promising approach: time-restricted eating, generally known as skipping breakfast.

Time-restricted eating limits the window of opportunity during which one may consume food to a certain length of time throughout the day, often anywhere from four to 12 hours. For instance, if you choose to consume all of your meals and snacks within a 10-hour window, ranging from 9 am to 7:00 pm, this represents an overnight fasting period. Evidence shows that brain function, glucose metabolism, and the healthy signaling of metabolic hormones are all improved by using this strategy.

In animal experiments aiming to replicate the effects of shift work, time-restricted feeding has previously been demonstrated to reduce the severity of depression and anxiety symptoms. Eating at specified times throughout the day has been an antidepressant impact in human studies. Eating every day may help minimize the risk of health problems, including obesity, diabetes, and heart disease. It is another benefit of eating on a normal schedule.

Our environment operates on a 24-hour cycle, and we have access to food and light sources at all times of the day and night. As a result, the influence that disrupted eating cycles have on mental health has become an essential concern for contemporary living. Incorporating eating rhythm therapy into clinical care might dramatically enhance people's quality of life as more research produces data measuring eating rhythms in persons with mood problems. It is crucial to enhance public education on approaches that are both accessible and economical to maintain good eating habits, particularly for the general population. It involves paying attention not just to the components of meals but also to the patterns of eating that occur throughout those meals. There will be enduring advantages for one's overall well-being if their eating cycles are aligned with the timetable of the Sun, and there is a possibility that this may have a protective impact against mental illness.

Mood Swings

If you have ever experienced the condition known as "hangry," you already know that a sufficiently empty stomach may give rise to emotions of impatience and rage. If you practice intermittent fasting for a sufficient amount of time, your mood will likely begin to change visibly.

Feeling grumpy? According to Susan Albers-Bowling, a psychotherapist at the Health Center and writer of Eating Mindfully for Hanger Management, this is due to falling blood glucose levels and "an increase in cortisol, the hormone cortisol, which occurs when individuals get too hungry."

According to Ansari, the reductions in blood sugar, followed by subsequent surges while "feasting," may be particularly dangerous for those with diabetes since they can induce a loss of control over blood glucose and impact the amount of diabetic medicine and insulin that is required.

Combative? That also makes perfect sense. In addition, there is a hormone known as neuropeptide Y that causes individuals to become more hostile when they are really hungry. This behavior has been traced back to the time of the cave dwellers when the only way to feed was to win a battle or your food.

Anxiety

The higher your cortisol levels are and the longer they have been there, the greater the likelihood that you will feel stressed. Some evidence suggests that engaging in behaviors associated with limited dietary intake might increase the stress hormone cortisol. It, in turn, can induce changes in one's food choices, cravings, and mood.

Since elevated cortisol levels have been related to increased fat accumulation, intermittent fasting can be counterproductive if your goal is to reduce your body fat percentage.

Tiredness

Although one preliminary study revealed that practicing intermittent fasting may help you have a better night's sleep, other research suggests that doing so is more likely to make sleep difficulties more probable. According to research in the journal Science and Nature of Sleep, fasting may reduce the amount of rapid eye movement (REM) sleep, which is the deepest and most restorative kind of sleep. It is because the body experiences increased cortisol and glucose during fasting.

You could stop eating several hours before bed, depending on your intermittent fasting technique. It can benefit you since eating right before bedtime is not good for your health and can lead to weight gain, acid reflux, excessive gas, and trouble sleeping. However, according to Michal Hertz, having an empty stomach that is rumbling in discomfort might make sleeping and staying asleep very difficult.

And let's face it, a good amount of sleep is necessary for your general mental health: Alterations in the way you sleep, the quality of your sleep, and the length of time you sleep may all contribute to feelings of exhaustion and alter your mood the subsequent day.

Loneliness

Social interactions with family and friends that include food may be difficult if you cannot consume food during certain periods. According to the American Psychological Association findings, not spending enough time with friends may result in loneliness and social isolation, which quickly snowball into feelings of melancholy. Moreover,

According to the National Anorexia Nervosa Association, people who struggle with anorexia have fewer friends, fewer social activities, and less social support than those who do not have an eating disorder. One of the hallmark symptoms of anorexia is skipping social occasions because of dietary restrictions.

Risk of Eating Disorder

Both Albers-Bowing, as well as Hertz believes that the stringent rules associated with intermittent fasting regarding when it is permissible to eat and when it is not permissible to eat could be problematic for a person who does have a history of the eating problem or who may be at risk for developing one in the future.

Anorexia involves, at its most fundamental level, imposing limitations, and rigid rules on one's eating habits, ignoring feelings of hunger and richness, and having burdening thoughts about food. All of these characteristics have the potential to be perpetuated and magnified by intermittent fasting (IF). In the same vein, are you familiar with the term orthorexia? It is an eating disorder trying to pass itself off as healthful eating.

According to Ansari, the diet also may generate a fear of losing control over food and overeating on days when there are no dietary restrictions to follow. Both of these are indicators that someone may have a problem with binge eating. One study discovered that women who cut their intake of calories by 70 percent for 4 days and afterward ate "normally" for four for a minimum of 4 weeks had a little more wanting to eat thoughts, enhanced fear of lack of control, and a regular tendency to overindulge during non-restricted periods of hunger. It resulted from the women eating for a minimum of 4 weeks. According to Albers-Bowling, IF may also be used to mask the symptoms of an underlying eating problem.

If you discover that you cannot remove the thought of food from your mind or that you are eating more of it than you normally would if you've not fast, then it is likely that intermittent fasting is not for you. If you have a past binge eating or a bad connection with food, experts suggest avoiding intermittent fasting entirely. It is because it may exacerbate these issues. According to Hertz, intermittent fasting (IF) may hurt anyone's relationship to food, but it is particularly dangerous for people who have a background of disordered eating. They have a larger propensity to use the regulations and limits to aid and intensify their eating problem.

Impact on Cognitive Thinking

Research has shown that being without food for an extended time might cause you to generate more snap judgments and focus less on the long term.

When you go without food for an extended period, you also cause changes in the chemicals that are available in your brain. Therefore, avoiding meals that raise your serotonin level might cause your brain to produce less of the chemical that makes you feel good, making you more impulsive. Consider the following before making any choices on food:

In the meantime, additional research conducted on mice and published in the Article In the journal of Scientific Studies in Biosciences suggests that fasting may increase tiers of certain neurotransmitters, including serotonin, and strengthen memory and learning. There is, without a doubt, data that contradicts itself, and this is true of a significant portion of the most recent studies on intermittent fasting and the claims made in this essay. Do you have a migraine? Same. Despite our best efforts, there are still many aspects of IF that we do not fully comprehend at this time.

Chapter 6: Stress-Free Recipes Eating Plan

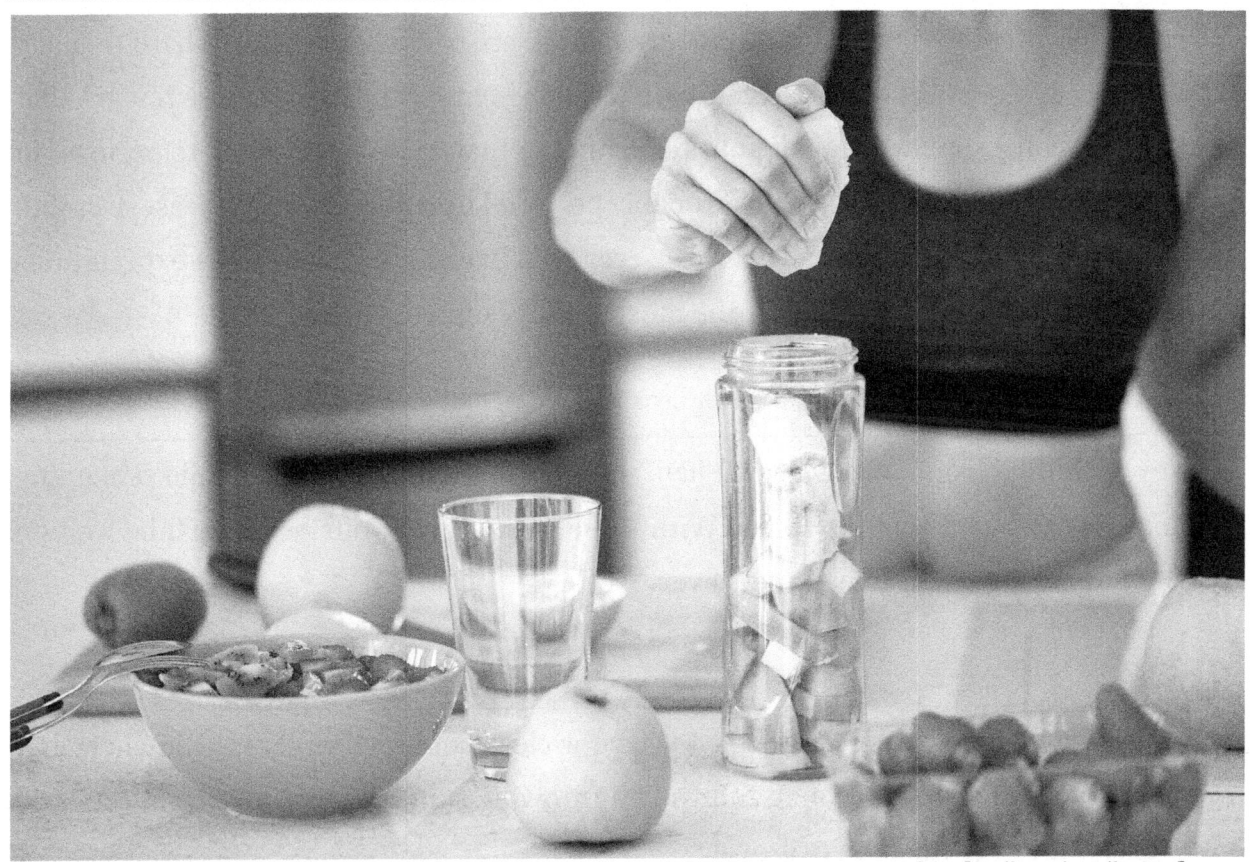

Never in human history has the process of preparing food appeared to be "easier." We have easy access to a diverse selection of foods in supermarkets, an abundance of items labeled as "convenience" meals, technologies that help every task more quickly, and enough recipes to last a lifetime. But despite this, many of us still consider setting the table for supper to be a stressful errand. People who are constantly on the go and under a lot of stress are more likely to put on weight because they eat at fast-food restaurants and dine out more frequently. This makes sense; if you've had a long day filled with errands and other commitments, you might not have the chance to attend home and prepare a meal from scratch.

But eating healthily at home, where the food you prepare is typically far better for you. Cooking at home could save you money, which can, in turn, reduce the amount of stress you feel by putting you under financial pressure. In other words, cooking at home can reduce stress. After a hard day at work, it could seem like a daunting effort to come home to cook something nutritious or novel, but it's easier than you might think to do so. Why? The selections presented to us in this modern culture are overwhelming. It is hard to make decisions because we become paralyzed by indecision. Some people might also remark that eating has become somewhat analogous to fashion in that we feel pressured to perform in unrealistic ways. Camping and hiking probably provided us with some of the least stressful, easiest-to-prepare, and tastiest meals we've ever had. Because our options as expectations were more restricted, we could make the most of the resources we had.

Get Rid Of Tension In The Kitchen

The key is to establish habits that will help us become more productive while remaining inside our established comfort zones. With these steps under your belt, you'll be well on your way to having stress-free dinners every week.

Organize Your Kitchen

It may sound like an impossible idea to have a clean and well-organized kitchen, but investing some time going through things and throwing some of them away will save you hours every day once the project is over.

- Make sure you check the refrigerator and the pantry. Throw away any stale food that you haven't eaten in a while. Please note any items you forget you had in the kitchen and try to include them in the forthcoming meals.
- Organize draw and cabinets in your home. It is not essential to finish the task all at once; rather, it can be incorporated into the weekly cleaning routine in stages, one cabinet or drawer at a time.
- Only keep the necessary things and those you use frequently. Place a box labeled "garage sale" in your basement and use it to store any equipment, dishes, silverware, or other items you haven't used in the past twelve months. If you can't bring yourself to get rid of items, try to find a location to store them that isn't the kitchen.

- Update your equipment. Cooking can be made much simpler and more enjoyable with the addition of certain kitchen appliances, such as a food processor, a stick blender, or a nice set of knives.
- Free of dirt and debris. A work atmosphere with clean seats and clear spaces is easier and more inspirational to be in. Put ornamental objects on shelves or in other rooms and instruct everyone in the household not to throw their keys, wallets, money, and bags on the kitchen counter.

Prepare A Strategy And A Plot

Even while it can seem impossible to "find the time to plan," doing so will keep you both time and anxiety in the long run. It is also possible for you to save money.

- Create a plan for your meals for the week. This can be completed in as little as ten minutes once per week. Consider any ingredients that are getting low on stock.
- Make sure you plan at least once daily that may be used as the foundation for another dinner the following night. For example, you can make chicken risotto with chicken burritos with the leftovers from roasting a chicken and then serving it.
- Include in your strategy the use of any equipment, such as crockpots or bread machines, that you already own. These can make cooking easier, saving both time and money.
- Compile a list of your go-to meals, and keep this list close at hand. When there are so many cookbooks and periodicals to choose from, it's easy to lose track of your go-to recipes. It would help if you noted each dish that turns out well as you eat it. Put this note on the refrigerator as a reminder to keep it handy so that you will never run out of ideas.
- To reduce stress, eat meals that you are familiar with regularly. Nothing is more reassuring than turning to a tried-and-true favorite.
- Create a key of items to buy at the store. Include essentials such as flour, cereal, bread, milk, tea, coffee, herbs, and spices in your shopping list. Include other frequently found components in pantries, such as canned beans, sauces, canned fruit, jams, and

chutneys. Please provide a list of your preferred fresh fruits and vegetables, dairy products, and typical cuts of meat, fish, or poultry. The lines should be left open for other objects. Produce numerous copies by the printing or photocopying them, and post one of them on the refrigerator or another convenient location each week. Appropriately mark your list each time you either completely run through an item or come dangerously close.

- Arrange the items on your checklist in the same manner as your grocery store. If you must go through the produce part first, organize your templates so that the produce section comes first.
- Shop shrewdly
- Limit your shopping to once every week. You lose both time and money on each outing to the store. If you spend less time shopping, you'll have more time to spend in the kitchen or doing other activities. If you want to avoid lines and angry customers, go shopping outside peak hours.
- Don't deviate from your list.
- Shopping while hungry is not a good idea. This may influence your decisions and cause you to put items in your shopping cart that you do not require. Consider purchasing in large quantities if things on your overview are now on sale; purchasing them in large quantities to stock your pantry could save you money.

Be A Wise Cook

- Make sure everyone is comfortable. Stick to the foods and preparation methods you are comfortable with to maintain your confidence. Hang your head high when you carry on the family custom of cooking Nana's and Mum's dishes if they are some of your favorites. Extend yourself only when you genuinely feel like it; don't do it to keep up with the Joneses, appease other people, or win people over.
- Make use of our chart titled "lunch in minutes." Keep the components for a few dishes on hand for those evenings when time is short, you are exhausted, or you need a vacation from cooking.

- Make effective use of your time. Set aside five minutes there in the morning to fill your slow cooker and learn how to use it. Make use of the pre-set function on both your oven and bread machine. Defrost any frozen products that you might require in advance.
- Set aside sometime on the weekend or one night of the week to do all of your cooking in advance. Doubling a recipe requires a small amount of additional work, but it can result in a stress-free evening off throughout the following week. You may prepare several boneless chicken wings at once and then use them in the dinners over the following two days; you can cut them up and add them to cooked pasta, slice and place them on salads or pizzas. Alternately, you may combine the chicken stock and a can of maize to make a delicious chicken & corn soup.
- Make basic recipes in large quantities and store them in the freezer. Simple recipes like mince may be swiftly transformed into various mouthwatering dishes in a short amount of time.
- Develop a cordial relationship with your slow cooker. Remove the layer of dust that has accumulated, and put it to good use. The number of foods that can be prepared in a slow cooker is practically unbounded, and some examples include soups, casseroles, and corned beef. The preparation of a meal that, in most cases, results in sufficient leftovers for yet another meal requires little more than a few hours of actual labor.
- You shouldn't be scared to stray somewhat from the instructions given in a recipe. If you only possess sunflower oil on hand, but the recipe calls for canola oil, you can use sunflower oil instead. Raisins can be used in sultanas, figs can be used in place of prunes, and oregano can be used in place of mixed herbs. These substitutions can be made without affecting the final product's success. If you don't have any spaghetti sauce on hand, you can use a can of beans that have been pureed with a little bit of tomato sauce added. If you are a competent cook, you will likely make substitutions and be creative in the kitchen; it is doubtful that you will ruin a recipe.
- Exercise extreme caution when you bake. A note of caution: the ratios of flour, fluid, eggs, sugar, and oil in baked products like cakes, muffins, and other bakery items are very specific. It is hazardous to change the proportions of something unless you have

prior experience doing so. You are nonetheless free to use brown sugar in place of white, spreads with a lower fat content in place of butter, and trim milk in place of full-fat cream.

- Make one night a week 'MasterChef night'. Holding a cooking contest might be fun to give oneself a night off. Participating members of the household, such as roommates, partners, or children of an appropriate age, should take turns coming up with innovative new dishes to amaze the rest of the family. Include award-winning recipes on your list of favorite meals.

Advice From The Experts

When you get into the routine of preparing more nutritious meals at home, you might discover that you can whip up something in about fifteen minutes or less. If it continues to appear to be an intolerably tense situation, the following are some additional suggestions that will make it simpler:

- Get Things Ready: Before you turn in for the night, make sure that everything is ready for the following day. This way, it will only take a minute, and you will spend those few minutes when you aren't famished and attempting to get dinner on the table. This way, it will only take a couple of minutes.
- Enlist Help: Delegate some of the labor if you've had a spouse and children. Mopping up after dinner won't seem daunting if you know that you will have assistance with it. Put on some tunes for some lighthearted competition and see how much you can get done as a group before the conclusion of a song or two.
- Make Use of Paper: For individuals who truly want to minimize time spent cleaning up, throwaway plates and cutlery are always options. Suppose the concept of just throwing away the trash when you are finished eating can make a difference between eating out at a restaurant and eating at home. In that case, you should give it a shot even though it is not as environmentally friendly. You would be able to save more money than the cost of both the plates compared to what you'd have paid, regardless of if you ate out.

Make Use Of A Service That Delivers Recipe Boxes

Sign up for a service that sends you pre-measured ingredients and detailed instructions along with a recipe box if you enjoy becoming a home cook but despises the actual tasks of shopping and meal preparation. These services will save you time in the kitchen and a trip to the grocery store. To utilize these services, you will need to go online, select the number of people and the amount of meals you want each week, and then pay the appropriate charge. After that, you select your meals from a list of delicious and nutritious options already prepared for you.

The application will give you a box that is stocked with all of the fresh, pre-portioned ingredients that you will require for each meal and detailed instructions on making the dish. Prepare the ingredients, combine them, and then cook them, and you're done! The majority of these meal delivery services include good selections for you. They typically have fixed portions to aid in reducing the amount of food that is wasted. In addition, some establishments provide you the opportunity to personalize your meal by providing gluten-free, macronutrient, or vegetarian options.

Although recipe boxes could appear to be an expensive choice at first glance when the cost of your typical grocery shopping trip is factored in and the possibility that food will be thrown out, you might save money by purchasing them. In the hope that they do, these pointers will better enable you to break out of the cycle of eating out and begin a new eating plan that is healthier. Your stress levels do not need to increase, and both your body and your checkbook will be grateful if you avoid doing so.

Chapter 7: Hidden Power Of Intermittent Fasting To Control Mood, Anxiety, And Depression

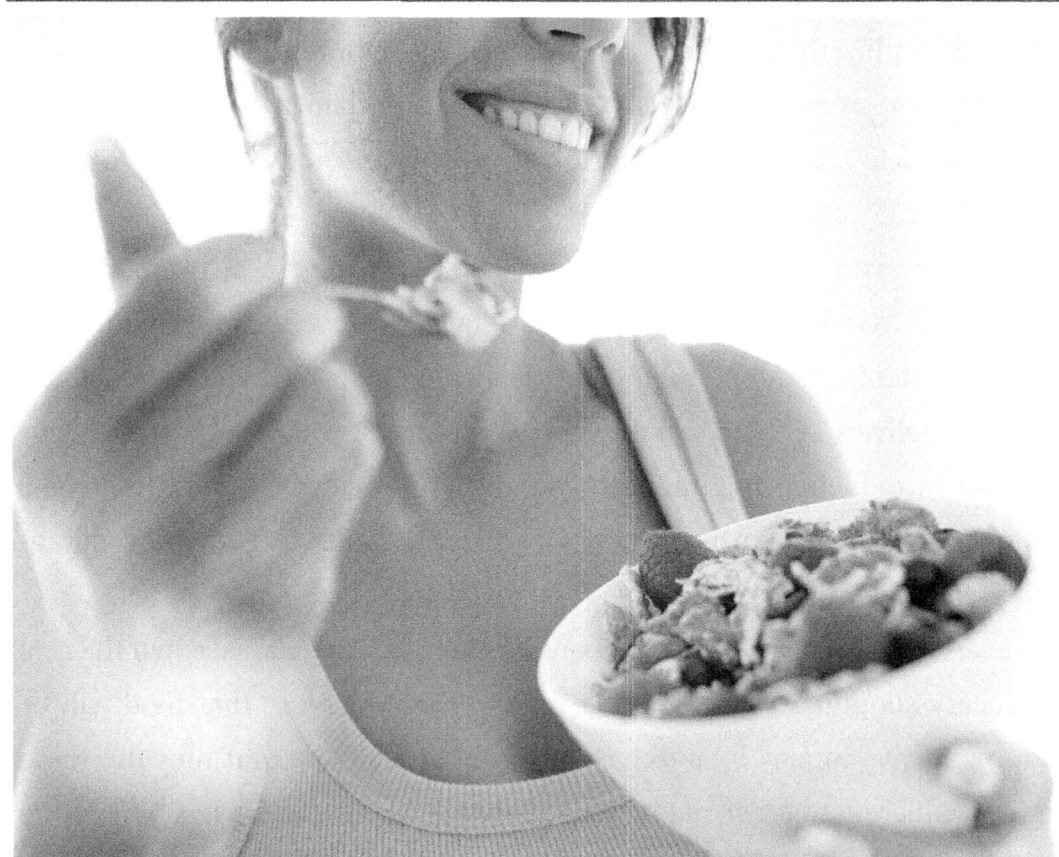

There is evidence that therapies that include fasting are useful in reducing symptoms of stress, anxiety, and depression. On the other side, there hasn't been any quantitative study done up to this point. This study aimed to investigate whether fasting therapies related to increased or reduced levels of weariness and energy and Methods. In all studies, individuals were considered for inclusion in the quantitative analysis. Results. After restricting our analysis to randomized controlled studies with minimal risk of bias, we concluded that those who participated in fasting had decreased levels of anxiety, depression, & body mass index when compared to the control group without experiencing an increase in tiredness. No publication bias nor heterogeneity could be found concerning these findings. Even in individuals diagnosed with type 2 diabetes, these therapies were risk-free. Conclusions. These findings need to be interpreted with a disclaimer in mind. These are early data, but they are promising, and it looks that fasting is a risk-free strategy. Due to a lack of applicable/appropriate data, we cannot provide a recommendation on whether fasting intervention is superior to the others. No research was conducted on psychiatric populations; nevertheless, further trials must be conducted on these groups since they would be suitable candidates for fasting therapies.

Anxiety and depression disorders are the top causes of disability & loss of product life year among persons younger than 40 years old all over the globe. Antidepressants are the therapy of choice for these illnesses; however, they are only helpful in around half of the patients and often come with a host of unwanted side effects. The present study faces a significant obstacle in the form of a huge challenge in identifying novel pathophysiological pathways to create individualized therapies for various conditions and enhance the benefit-to-risk ratio. With the recent findings on the microbiome & its function in both anxiety and depression, one of these novel routes, known as the gut-brain axis, has aroused much attention among medical researchers. The study of psych nutrition has emerged in tandem with the discoveries of the preventative influence that eating a healthy, anti-inflammatory diet may have on the development of depression and the efficacy of omega-3 fatty acids, among other nutrients, in the treatment of anxiety & depression.

Some clinical studies were conducted in the 1990s and 2000s to investigate the impact of therapeutic fasting on depression and anxiety, but the findings were inconsistent, and no control group did not include fasting. In parallel, therapies that include fasting are simultaneously gaining more and more popularity among the public. People who go through these fasts almost universally report feeling mentally better because of the experience.

Reducing the total number of hours spent eating each day is the essential component of an intermittent fast. Fasting once or twice a week, fasting for 12 to 18 hours per day, or any combination of these are all acceptable intermittent fasting. Interest in the potentially beneficial effects that intermittent fasting might have on mood has increased. Fasting may be an effective treatment for reducing depression symptoms by increasing weight reduction, which relates to being overweight or obese, associated with greater depression.

According to research conducted on rodents and humans, intermittent fasting may transition glucose metabolism towards ketone metabolism, causing anti-inflammatory, anti-oxidative, and stress resistance benefits. These studies have demonstrated that this may result in weight reduction. Microbiota abnormalities and intestinal inflammation may be improved by fasting. It is accomplished by reducing the consumption of inflammatory meals and the amount of blood flow allocated to digesting. The advancement of fasting therapies may be hampered by concerns about the acceptability and safety of intermittent fasting. It is unknown whether therapies, including fasting, might lead to decreased energy or increased weariness. It is an important subject because weariness is a prevalent sign of depression. It is common practice to combine intermittent fasting with calorie restriction; however, it is not certain which of these two methodologies is the most successful in alleviating the symptoms of anxiety and depression. It is one of the many questions that still need to be answered. To answer this issue, researchers conducted a randomized controlled experiment that compared the effects of calorie restriction in patients with type 2 diabetes who either had or did not have a 14-hour eating restriction. The scientists concluded that both courses of treatment were related to reduced symptoms of depression. It leads them to advise that calorie restriction should be explored among fasting therapies. This systematic review & meta-analysis was conducted to determine whether fasting therapies are beneficial in reducing stress, anxiety, and depression. Confirming that these therapies were also helpful in lowering body mass index was the secondary aim, as did determining whether these interventions were related to increased or reduced fatigue/energy levels.

Can Intermittent Fasting Boost Mood?

These days, Intermittent Fasting(IF) is all the rage, and it has been the focus of numerous films, blogs, and publications. The claims made for this mode of consumption appear more like those of a late-night television commercial that is too good to be true. The steak knives are free!) if it weren't for a considerable body of data demonstrating that restricting calories and engaging in brief periods of fasting sometimes may have major impacts on the body, this theory wouldn't hold up.

It has been shown that intermittent fasting when practiced in humans, can

- Cause a reduction in body weight
- Increase your body's responsiveness to insulin.
- Lower your blood pressure Lower the risk of inflammation
- Reduce the amounts of hormones that have been related to a higher risk of cancer, particularly IGF-1.

Famously, it's been demonstrated to dramatically extend the lifespan of animals (by twofold in yeast and by thirty percent in rodents) and to enhance the prognosis of several different types of cancer. Additionally, it's been shown to increase cellular stress tolerance in the heart and the muscle.

However, the impact of intermittent fasting upon Woody Allen's absolute favorite organ, the brain, has not garnered as much study as the effects of the fasting pattern on other organs. In addition, the review that the NIH conducted describes the current state of our knowledge about the effects that Intermittent Fasting(IF) has on the brain.

How Food Impacts Mood?

There is an overlap in the brain circuits responsible for regulating mood and eating, even though the underlying practices/processes have not been fully elucidated. Dopamine is a neurotransmitter that plays a significant role in regulating mood, energy, and enjoyment. Additionally, digestive hormones influence dopamine. Patients suffering from depression and bipolar illness have levels of dopamine that are not usual. It is believed that alterations in eating cycles might lead to mental problems.

Inconsistent eating patterns have even been hypothesized to contribute to mood disorders' many factors. For instance, people who suffer from depression or bipolar illness often have disrupted internal cycles and inconsistent mealtimes. Both factors contribute considerably to the worsening of mood symptoms. In addition to this, shift workers, who often have erratic eating habits, have been shown to exhibit higher rates of sadness and anxiety compared with the general population. Despite the evidence to the contrary, monitoring eating cycles is not now a regular component of therapeutic therapy in most psychiatric settings.

Why Does Fasting Affect Brain Health And Mood?

The concept of hormesis, which states that a modestly negative stimulation might guard against a future more severe shock, is one of the most intriguing theories. In animal studies, intermittent fasting has been shown to result in higher cognition neurotrophic factor, which is thought to play an imperative role in the effect that antidepressants have, as well as an increase in neurogenesis, enhanced synaptic plasticity, and an improvement in the animal's ability to tolerate stress. In other words, it is plausible that intermittent fasting may be making these rats' brains more robust and resistant to damage.

Other hypotheses have investigated the effects of fasting on the metabolism of serotonin, the improvement of sleep quality, and the impact of ketone bodies.

Mental Function

When you don't eat for a period, your body eliminates waste products and toxins from the circulation of blood and lymph, which clears your mind and makes it simpler to think. When you don't eat for a period, the brain is free to use the energy that would ordinarily go into breaking down Food.

Because your body needs time to readjust, you probably won't notice any changes to your mental state until after you've been fasting for a few days. At the start of the investigation, you can experience some pain or discomfort, such as headaches. But when your body has rid itself of toxins, the brain will have access to a cleaned bloodstream, which will result in more distinct ideas, an improved ability to remember things, and an improvement in the understanding of other senses.

Optimized Eating

The question now is, what could be done to make the most of our eating rhythms? We came across one approach that shows promise during our investigation: time-restricted eating, called intermittent fasting.

Time-restricted eating limits the window of opportunity during which one may consume

Food for a certain length of time throughout the day, often anywhere from four to 12 hours. For instance, if you choose to consume all your meals and snacks within a 10-hour window, ranging from 9:00 a.m. - to 7:00 p.m., this represents an overnight fasting period. Evidence shows that by using this strategy, energy metabolism, brain function, and the healthy signaling of metabolic hormones are all improved.

In animal experiments aiming to replicate the effects of shift work, time-restricted feeding has previously been demonstrated to reduce the severity of depression and anxiety symptoms. Eating at specified times throughout the day has been an antidepressant impact on human studies. Eating simultaneously every day may help minimize the risk of health problems, including diabetes, obesity, and cardiovascular disease. It is another benefit of eating on a regular schedule.

Our environment operates on a 24-hour cycle, and we have access to food and light sources at all times of the day & night. As a result, the influence that disrupted eating cycles have on mental health has become an essential concern for contemporary living. Incorporating eating rhythm therapy into clinical care might dramatically enhance people's quality of life as more research produces data measuring eating rhythms in persons with mood problems. It is crucial to enhance public education on approaches that are both accessible and economical to maintain good eating habits, particularly for the general population. It involves paying attention not just to the components of meals but also to the patterns of eating that occur throughout those meals. There will be enduring advantages for one's overall well-being if their eating cycles are aligned with the timetable of the Sun, and there is a possibility that this may have a protective impact against mental illness.

Chapter 8: Healthy Eating Tips And Tricks

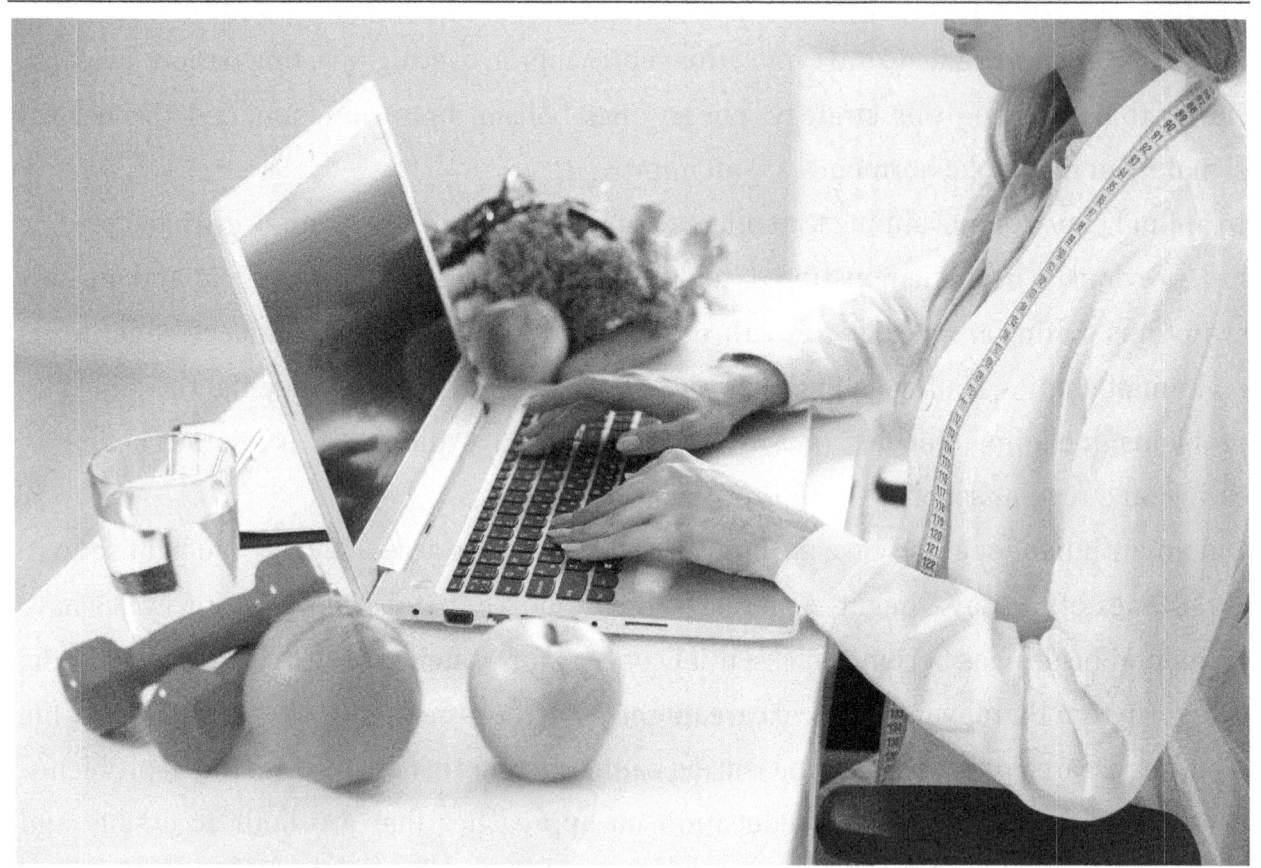

Women have special dietary demands. By maintaining a healthy diet throughout your life, you may curb cravings, maintain a healthy weight, increase your energy level, and feel and look you're very best.

Maintaining a nutritious diet may be challenging for any woman who is simultaneously juggling the responsibilities of her family, career, or education, not to mention dealing with the pressure from the media to behave and appear a particular way. On the other hand, consuming the appropriate foods may help you keep a healthy weight, enhance your mood, and give you more energy, but it can also support you as you go through the many seasons of a woman's life.

As women, many are usually prone to overlooking our nutritional requirements, which might have negative consequences. You could believe that you don't have enough time to eat healthily or that you're used to placing your family's requirements ahead of your own need. Or, it's possible that you're attempting to maintain a strict diet, one that deprives your body of essential nutrients and leaves you feeling irritable, hungry, and drained of energy.

Dietary research too often ignores the requirements that are unique to women. In nutritional research, male volunteers are often used since their hormone levels are much more consistent and reliable; consequently, the findings might sometimes be irrelevant or even deceptive to the requirements of women. All these factors may contribute to significant deficiencies in your regular diet.

Varying Nutritional Requirements Of Women

While they are young, boys' and girls' nutritional requirements are comparable. However, as puberty sets in, women start to acquire dietary needs that are specific to them. And as we get older, our bodies undergo more physiological and hormonal changes, which causes our nutritional requirements to fluctuate over time. Because of this, our diets must adapt over time to accommodate these shifting requirements.

Even though women typically need fewer calories than men do, our requirements for several minerals and vitamins are much greater. Because of the hormonal shifts that occur during menstruation, pregnancy, and menopause, women are at a greater risk of developing anemia, osteoporosis, and brittle bones. As a result, they need to consume more nutrients like iron, potassium, magnesium, Vit D, and vitamin B9 to protect themselves from these conditions.

Why vitamins and minerals aren't enough on their own

It was common practice for women to take vitamins and other dietary supplements to compensate for dietary deficiencies. However, even though supplements may be a helpful defense against occasional vitamin deficits, they are not capable of compensating for an unhealthy diet that is not balanced.

If you want to make sure that the food you consume provides you with all the essential nutrients, you should strive for a diet that is high in fresh fruit and vegetables, high-quality protein, and healthy fats, yet low in processing, fried, or sugary foods.

Calcium is essential for healthy bones throughout one's life.

Calcium is essential for some bodily processes, including the development of strong bones and teeth, the maintenance of bone density with age, the maintenance of normal heart rhythm, and the maintenance of a healthy brain system. Problems with one's mood, such as irritation, anxiety, sadness, and inability to sleep, may be caused by a lack of calcium or can worsen these conditions. If you do not consume adequate calcium from your food, your body will draw calcium levels to maintain proper cell function. It might result in brittle bones or osteoporosis in the long run. Because osteoporosis affects women at a higher rate than men, it is essential to receive adequate calcium and magnesium plus vitamin D to maintain healthy bones. It is especially crucial for women.

What are your recommended daily intakes of calcium, mg, and vitamin D?

Calcium has a recommended daily requirement of 1,000 milligrams (mg) that should be met by adult women between the ages of 19 and 50, according to the United States Department of Agriculture (USDA). The maximum daily dose that women should take over 50 is 1,200 mg. The consumption of dairy products, green leafy vegetables, certain fish, cereals, tofu, broccoli, and summer squash are excellent ways to receive your daily dose of calcium. The maximum dose that your body can process at any moment is 500 milligrams, and there is no advantage to taking more than the suggested daily quantity.

Magnesium: Magnesium enhances the body's ability to take calcium from the blood and deposit it into the bone. Your body is unable to use calcium if it is not there. According to the USDA, the recommended magnesium intake ranges from 320 to 400 milligrams per day. Vegetables that are leafy green and dark in color, summer squash, broccoli, fish, cucumber, black beans, celery, and a wide range of seeds are excellent sources.

Vitamin D: Calcium must be properly metabolized, and vitamin D is essential to this process. Aim for a daily intake of 600 IU (international units). Vitamin D may be obtained by exposure to the Sun for around half an hour and from certain foods and beverages, including cod, eggs, salmon, shrimp, and milk that has been fortified with vitamin D.

Diet Tips for PSM Symptoms

For the week, or please do tell your period, it is common to experience changing hormones, which may cause symptoms such as bloating, cramps, and exhaustion. Your food has the potential to play a significant part in reducing this and many other symptoms of premenstrual syndrome (PMS).

- Consume meals that are rich in both iron and zinc. Some women find that eating items that assist reduce the symptoms of premenstrual syndromes, such as red meat, meat, eggs, leafy green vegetables, and dried fruit, may be beneficial.
- Increase the amount of calcium in your diet. Several studies have emphasized the importance calcium-rich foods have in alleviating the symptoms of premenstrual syndrome (PMS), such as milk, yogurt, cheese, and vegetables with leafy greens.
- Steer clear of trans fats, deep-fried meals, and sugar. All of them are inflammatory, and inflammation is a known PMS trigger.
- Eliminating salt from your diet might help reduce bloating. Avoiding snack foods, frozen meals, and processed foods may significantly improve water retention and bloating symptoms in those who have this tendency.
- Watch out for allergic reactions to certain foods. Food sensitivities can present themselves with premenstrual syndrome (PMS). Dairy products and wheat are two of the most common allergens. Remove the possible offending food from your diet and observe whether your symptoms improve.
- Stop drinking coffee and alcoholic beverages. Both may make PMS symptoms worse. Therefore, it is best to avoid them when experiencing this phase of your cycle.
- Consider vitamin supplements. Taking regular multivitamins or a supplement containing magnesium, b Vitamins, and vitamin E might help reduce cramps for some women. It may also be the case with taking a multivitamin. However, dietary supplements are not just a suitable replacement for a nutritious and well-rounded diet. Consuming foods rich in the vitamins and minerals your body requires will always provide the best results.

- To alleviate cramping, take some essential fatty acids. It has been shown that omega-3 fatty acids may aid in the relief of cramps. Try increasing the amount of fish and flaxseed you consume to see if it helps your PMS symptoms.

Dietary recommendations during pregnancy

To meet the nutritional requirements of your developing child with just roughly 300 more calories per day, you may continue your normal diet. However, it is normal for a woman to have weight gain throughout pregnancy, and continuing to breastfeed after delivery may be beneficial for the mother's weight reduction efforts.

Pregnancy diet tips

- Omega-3 fats are necessary for the normal development of your kid's nervous system and early vision and breast milk production when the baby is born. Aim for two meals per week of chilled water fish like salmon, sardines, sardines, mackerel, or anchovies in your diet. Both sardines and seaweed are excellent sources of Omega-3 fatty acids. However, most people agree that eating sardines is the healthiest and most environmentally friendly option.
- Stay away from alcoholic beverages. The infant should not be exposed to any quantity.
- Caffeine, associated with an increased risk of complications and may interfere with the body's ability to absorb iron, should be consumed in much smaller amounts.
- Instead of a few big meals, you should eat several smaller meals more often. It will aid in preventing morning sickness and minimize the severity of heartburn.
- Pregnant women need to exercise caution regarding meals that might potentially hurt them. These include albacore tuna, stingray, tilefish, king mackerel, soft cheeses, sashimi, deli meats, fresh sprouts, and other types of fish with high mercury amounts.
- In addition, your baby's growing brain and neurological system need enough high-quality protein. Instead of depending only on red meat as a source of protein, consider including high-quality proteins like those found in fish, poultry, dairy products, and plant-based foods.

Breastfeeding diet tips

Maintaining a calorie intake that is greater than usual can assist your body in producing milk at a consistent rate.

- There is a greater need for good protein sources and calcium during breastfeeding than at other times. To maintain milk production, nursing mothers need around 20 more grams of high-quality protein per day than before they were pregnant.
- If your doctor has not instructed you differently, taking prenatal vitamins and supplements while nursing is beneficial to you and your baby.
- Stay away from coffee, alcohol, and cigarettes. Avoid consuming alcohol and smoking cigarettes, and cut down on your use of caffeine. These recommendations are like those found in the section above.
- If your child has an allergic response, you may have to change the foods you eat. Some foods, such as cow's milk, eggs, bread, fish, and citrus, may trigger allergic reactions. If you cannot consume cow's milk due to an allergy, you may still consume calcium-rich foods that do not contain cow's milk. Some examples of these foods are kale, broccoli, and sardines.

Chapter 9: Exercise Combined With Fasting

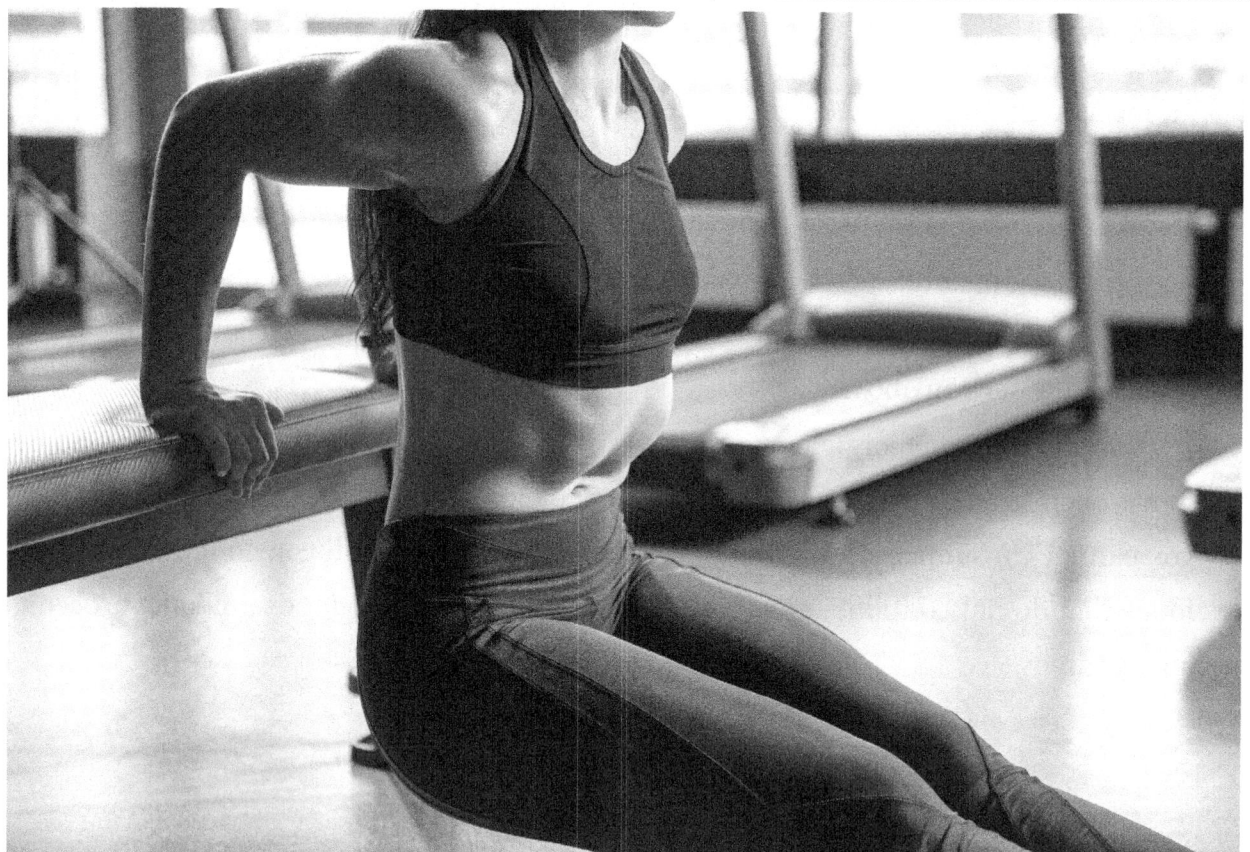

When you engage in physical activity while intermittent fasting, it can have a significant effect on your body, it will cause your body to behave differently to insulin and increase the amount of fat that your body burns in addition to lowering blood sugar levels, exercising while fasting boosts the production of synthetic testosterone and testosterone in the body as well as increasing the overall amount of these hormones produced. If you are a female, you require testosterone. Exercising fast speeds up the burning of fat, which increases the amount of weight that may be shed. You can accomplish your fitness objectives by following one of an astounding number of different meal plans that are available in today's modern wellness industry. However, this is a good reality that maintaining a healthy dietary pattern is only one piece of the puzzle determining your level of success. Combining a nutritious diet plan with consistent physical activity is essential to achieving the best possible outcomes. But is this plan suited for people who follow a variety of diets? Is it possible to combine intermittent fasting with physical activity? Will it not compromise your general health in any way? Have a look through the post to get the solutions to your questions.

Insulin Sensitivity

Insulin is a hormone that adjusts glucose, circulating in your bloodstream at any given time. Did you know that insulin also informs your body when and how to store fat and stimulates your muscles to sponge up sugar from the bloodstream and keep it for fuel when you have too much insulin in your system? The amount of glucose present in your blood increases whenever you consume food. When your blood glucose reaches a specific threshold, your body will produce insulin. Your muscle cells receive instructions from the insulin to remove glucose from your blood, subsequently stored as glycogen in the muscle cells. When your muscles reach their limit for sugar absorption, your body will store any remaining sugar as fat. Insulin resistance, also known as low insulin sensitivity, is a disorder that affects one in every three people in the United States. It means that your system is left with surplus glucose, which it has no choice but to store as body fat; nevertheless, your muscles do not receive the fuel they require to work at their highest potential. According to research, exercising while fasting can boost your insulin sensitivity, which is a significant benefit if your insulin levels are already within the usual range. If you have diabetes, it may be easier for you to lose weight, and your blood sugar levels will be better balanced. An increase in the human growth hormone is equivalent to a greater amount of muscle. The production of human growth hormone, often known as GH or HGH, is necessary for the body to repair and replace damaged tissue.

In addition to this, it assists in building muscle and the recovery process after exercise. After exercise, you should notice a rise in the amount of this essential hormone that your body produces. Insulin to human growth hormone should be administered specifically for the best possible health benefits. Exercising helps to enhance this ratio since it raises the amount of growth hormone (GH) present in your system. When insulin levels are high, growth hormone (GH) levels are low, and significant fat storage occurs in the body. When your growth hormone (GH) levels are low, your post-workout recovery may be slowed down, and it may be more complicated for you to pack on lean muscle. According to studies, engaging in physical activity while in a fasting condition can significantly raise the amounts of human growth hormone (HGH) in your body. If you practice fasting for shorter periods, you might not elicit a significant response; yet the consequences can still be spectacular.

Testosterone Levels Rise

It's a common misconception that testosterone only affects men. Men have higher testosterone levels, responsible for their deeper voices or facial hair. Although it is typically produced in lower quantities, females also produce testosterone. Therefore, why is increased testosterone a positive thing regarding physical activity? Because testosterone is essential for the growth of lean muscle. If your testosterone level is high, you'll have more stamina and store less fat in your body. If it's low, you'll store more of it.

Oxidation of Fat That Is More Efficient

According to the findings of several studies, intermittent fasting on its own can contribute to weight loss. When you participate in an activity, your body will first draw upon the easiest fuel source to reach, which is the glycogen stored in your muscles. After that, you'll put the extra glycogen stored in the liver. When all your glycogen stores are gone, you will switch to using fat as an energy source. When you exercise after fasting for such time (for example, halfway through the fasting period or immediately before your feeding period), your body will have already used up some of its stored glycogen, and in certain cases, it will have used up most of it. When there is no more glycogen for the body to use as an energy source, it begins to break down fat stores. The main point is: You may experience better results in your quest to reduce body fat if you exercise while you are fasting. Because of the changes occurring in your body's physiology, you may find that you can burn more fat and create more lean muscle.

The Numerous Advantages of Engaging in Physical Activity while Fasting

When you schedule your workouts during your fast, you will experience a large increase in the amount of fat burned. A study conducted in 2013 at Northumbia University discovered that if you exercise in the morning before eating breakfast, you can remove up to 20 percent more fat from your body. A key advantage of engaging in physical exercise while fasting is the development of lean muscle. Gaining more muscle mass will result in improved physical performance. In addition, you will expend more calories all day long, not just while you are working out. More fuel is required to maintain muscle than fat.

How Your Body Responds to Intermittent Fasting In conjunction with a wide range of physical activities Whether you perform aerobic activity alone or in conjunction with intermittent fasting, in a nutshell, however, some exercise, such as HIT, has induced an instantaneous increase in blood sugar. This is because HIIT causes your liver to release glycogen that it has been storing. If you already have diabetes, you need to pay close attention to your body, regardless of the type of physical activity you choose to engage in.

Why Going Out During Intermittent Fasting Might Not Be Effective

Exercising while fasting may have some beneficial effects, but there is also the possibility of having some adverse effects. Your blood sugar may drop to an unsafe level. The muscles in your body can take up glucose from your bloodstream more quickly and easily when you exercise because exercise increases insulin sensitivity. When you exercise while fasting, even less glucose is available for your legs to use, increasing the risk of passing out. There is also the possibility that your performance will suffer, especially if you are a professional athlete. According to the data that is now available, either there will be no change in performance, or it will decrease. According to a recent study, endurance athletes should avoid intense training while fasting. When considering whether fasting is the correct choice for you, it is important to think about your fitness goals. If losing fat is your primary objective, fasting may be effective. Either make sure you consume enough food throughout your eating window or experiment with a change in your eating plan if your goal is to put on muscle. In any case, give heed to any symptoms that your body displays when you work out.

When Should You Next Have a Meal?

When you eat, your body determines your goals for your workouts and the foods you consume during your eating periods. However, you should conduct cardio exercises before meals (this will allow you to get the most out of the fat-burning potential of the cardio) and save your HIIT workouts for one to two hours after meals for the greatest possible effects. Before you add fast exercise to the program, you need to get used to the habit of fasting first, and you shouldn't overdo it in the beginning. If you suddenly begin an overly active routine, it may cause low blood sugar. Therefore, look out for the symptoms of low blood sugar, which may include weakness, dizziness, "brain fog," fainting, and other symptoms. Try a starch drink if you feel faint or dizzy, and make sure you drink less on your next workout. Because it is very simple to become dehydrated during fasting, you mustn't leave. The risk of becoming dehydrated is multiplied when the calculation is factored into physical activity. Drink significantly more liquids than you believe you require and steer clear of sports drinks until your blood sugar lowers to an uncomfortably low level. So, is it possible to work out while you're fasting? Yes. Should you exercise even if you're fast? Absolutely, but be sure to pay attention to what your body needs. Fasting can be performed for various reasons, including religious or spiritual reasons, dietary reasons, or other health benefits. It is feasible to exercise even while on the IF diet safely. Although intermittent fasting (IF) and exercise may benefit weight loss, the evidence indicating that they are more efficient than the conventional, such as calorie restriction eating, is inconsistent. Both fasting and exercise can increase autophagy, a process that plays a role in cellular recycling, and may also have anti-aging effects.

On the other hand, folks who try intermittent fasting may discover that it hinders their ability to gain muscle and causes less success in the gym. If a person wants to put on muscle, they might want to investigate trying a different diet. There are a lot of different kinds of IF. No matter which option they go with, people should always be sure to plan their workouts ahead of time and think about how they can stay safe.

Chapter 10: Breakfast Recipes

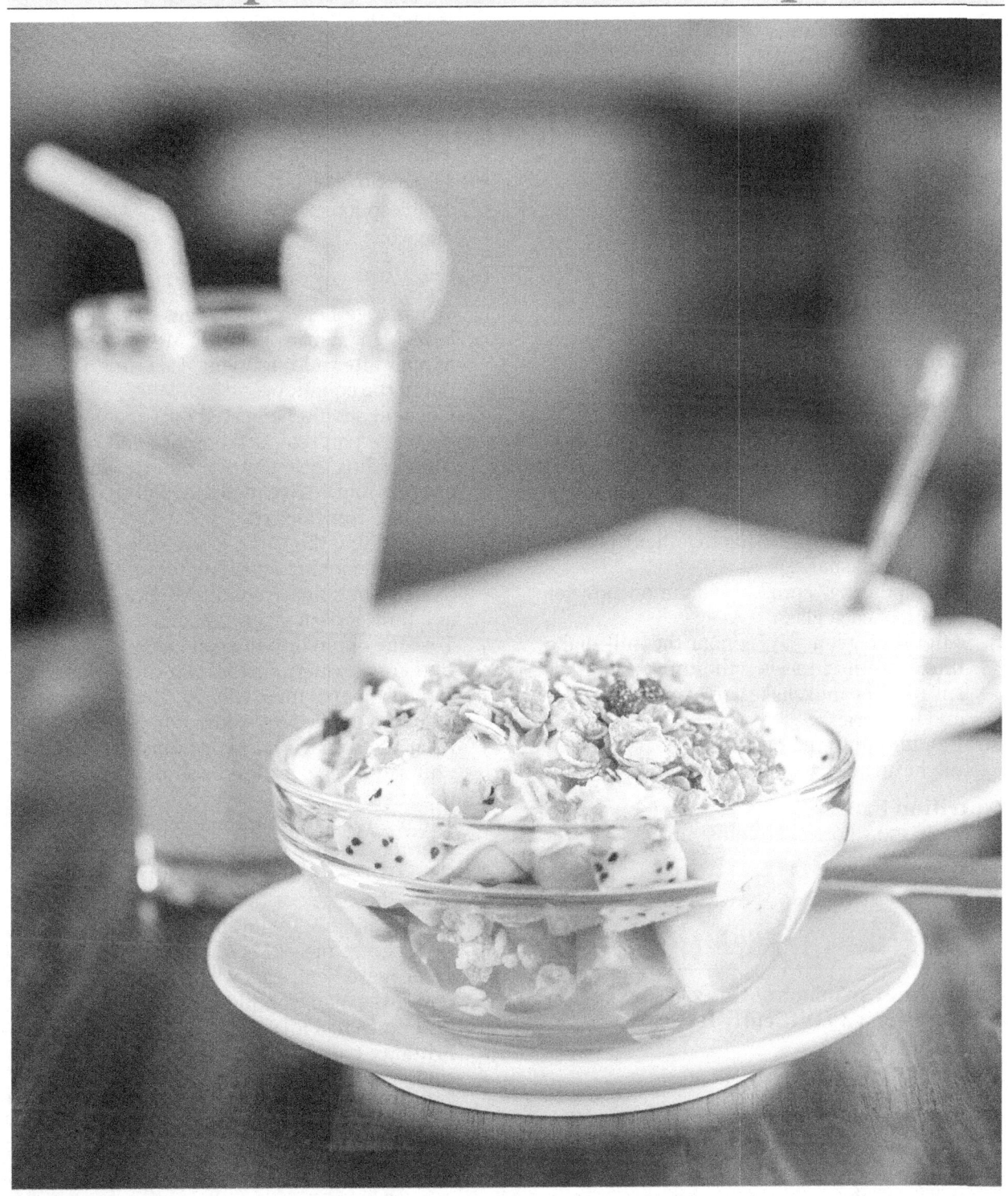

Keto Turmeric Milkshake

Prep Time: 5 minutes / **Cook Time:** 5 / **Servings:** 4 / **Difficulty level:** Moderate

Ingredients

- salt as required
- 1/2 teaspoon cinnamon 1 sugar-free pellets
- 1/2 teaspoon coconut oil
- 1 sugar-free pellet
- 1 teaspoon turmeric
- ice cubes as required
- 2 1/2 cup coconut milk

Instructions

1. In a blender or food processor, combine turmeric, ginger, sugar-free pellets, coconut milk, coconut oil, cinnamon, and a pinch of salt. Blend until smooth.
2. Shake all the ingredients together to create a thick milkshake.
3. After pouring, sprinkle cinnamon powder on top of each glass.
4. After that, get a glass & pour the milkshake into it until it reaches the top. After that, sprinkle the milkshake with some cinnamon and turmeric.
5. In addition to that, just before serving, you might include a couple of ice cubes.

Nutrition Facts
Calories: 150 calories, Proteins: 1.6g, Carbs: 12g, Fat: 35g.

Spinach Frittata

Prep Time: 20 minutes/ **Cook Time:** 10 / **Servings:** 4 / **Difficulty level:** Moderate

Ingredients

- 2 tablespoons chopped sun-dried tomatoes, optional
- 1/3 cup Parmesan cheese
- 9 large eggs
- 8 ounces (225g) or more fresh chopped spinach (or use baby spinach)
- 2 tablespoons milk
- 1/8 teaspoon pepper
- 1 medium onion
- 1/4 teaspoon salt
- 2 ounces (56g) of goat cheese
- 1 large clove of garlic, minced
- 2 tablespoons
- olive oil

Instructions

1. Whisk together the milk, eggs, and Parmesan cheese in a mixing bowl. Mix the salt and pepper after adding them. Take that variable out of the equation.
2. Olive oil should be heated over medium-high heat in a pan that is ovenproof and nonstick. After adding the onion, continue to simmer for another four to five minutes or until the onion becomes translucent.
3. After adding the garlic & sun-dried tomatoes, continue cooking for an additional minute (if using). The spinach should be added a handful at a time at each stage.
4. Toss the onion into the pan using tongs.
5. If there is room in the pan after the fresh spinach has begun to wilt, you may make room for more spinach by adding more to the pan. After the spinach has wilted, distribute it in a uniform layer over the base of the pan using the mixture.
6. The egg mixture/combination is then poured over the onion and spinach.
7. Using a spatula, carefully lift the mixture along the edges of the pan to make room for the egg mixture to flow underneath.
8. Goat cheese pieces should be sprinkled on top of the ingredients that will become the frittata.
9. Cover the pan completely after turning the heat down to a low level.
10. Frittatas typically take 10 to 13 minutes to cook on the stovetop or until all the ingredients outside the center are ready to eat. The center should keep its undulating shape.
11. Adjust the oven's temperature to broil. Put the dish you're going to bake in the upper third of

the oven. Place in the broiler for three minutes or until the top is golden brown.
12. Take out of the oven using oven mitts & lay aside for a few minutes to cool off.
13. When ready/geared up to serve, cut the loaf into wedges.

Nutrition Facts
Calories: 194.3 calories, Proteins: 12.6g, Carbs: 3.1g, Fat: 13.2g.

Fat-Burning Coconut Cookies

Prep Time: 35 /**Cook Time:** 25 /**Servings:** 5 /**Difficulty level:** Difficult

Ingredients

- 3 eggs
- ¼ cup almond flour
- 1 teaspoon almond milk
- 1 teaspoon baking powder
- ½ cup unsweetened coconut flakes
- ¼ cup almond flour
- 1 teaspoon almond milk
- ¾ cup granular sucralose sweetener
- ½ cup butter
- ½ tablespoon heavy cream
- 6 tablespoons coconut flour

Instructions

1. Whisk together the milk, eggs, and Parmesan cheese in a mixing bowl. Mix the pepper and salt after adding them. Take that variable out of the equation.
2. Olive oil should be heated over medium heat in a pan that is ovenproof and nonstick. After adding the onion, continue to simmer for another four to five minutes or until the onion becomes translucent.
3. After adding the garlic & sun-dried tomatoes, remaining cooking for an additional minute (if using), the spinach should be added a handful at each stage.
4. Toss the onion into the pan using tongs.
5. If there is room in the pan after the fresh spinach has begun to wilt, you may make room for more spinach by adding more to the pan. After the spinach has wilted, distribute it in a uniform layer over the base of the pan using the mixture.
6. The egg mixture/combination is then poured over the onion and spinach.
7. Using a spatula, carefully lift the mixture along the edges of the pan to make room for the egg mixture to flow underneath.
8. Goat cheese pieces should be sprinkled on top of the ingredients that will become the frittata.
9. Cover the pan completely after turning the heat down to a low level.
10. Frittatas typically take 10 to 13 minutes to cook on the stovetop or until all the ingredients outside of the center are ready to eat. (You may want to check the frittata more than once to see how it's setting.) The center should keep its undulating shape.
11. Adjust the oven's temperature to broil. Put the dish you're going to bake in the upper third of the oven. Place in the broiler for three minutes or until the top is golden brown.
12. Take out of the oven using oven mitts and lay aside for a few minutes to cool off.
13. When ready/gear up to serve, cut the loaf into wedges.

Nutrition Facts
Calories: 107 calories, Proteins: 4g, Carbs: 3g, Fat: 9g.

Baked Perfect Potato

Prep Time: 10/ **Cook Time:** 5 /**Servings:** /**Difficulty level:** Difficult

Ingredients

- 4 large russet potato
- canola oil
- kosher salt

Instructions

1. The oven/stove should be preheated(warmed) at 350 degrees Fahrenheit, and the racks should be placed in the top & lower thirds of the stove.
2. Before beginning to boil the potato (or potatoes), it is important to give them a thorough washing using a vigorous brush and water flowing cold.

3. After thoroughly drying the potato, use a standard fork to create 8 to 12 big trenches all over its surface. It will enable moisture to escape while the potato is being cooked.
4. Place the wet ingredients in the dish, and then use the oil to lightly cover them.
5. A little coating of kosher salt should be applied to the potato before it is placed directly on the inside(middle) rack of the stove/oven.
6. You may catch any drippings by placing a baking sheet on the lowest rack of the oven.
7. Bake for one hour or until the surface is golden brown and crisp, but the flesh on the inside is still soft.
8. First, use your forks to make a dot that extends from one end to the other; then, to serve, split the potato apart by pushing the two ends together.
9. It will open on its own in a moment. However, you need to be cautious since there will be a significant amount of steam.

Nutrition Facts
Calories: 161 calories, Protein: 4.3g, Carbs: 37g, Fat 0.2g.

Savory Oats and Roasted Veggies Bowl

Prep Time: 15 /**Cook Time:** 30 /**Servings:** /**Difficulty level**: Moderate

Ingredients

- 1 teaspoon divided black pepper
- 16-ounce bag butternut cubed squash
- 2 cup water
- 1 tablespoon olive oil
- ½ cup onion, chopped
- 8-ounce halved Brussels sprouts
- 2 strips of cooked crumbled turkey bacon
- 2 cup Old Quaker Fashioned Oats
- 1 teaspoon divided salt,
- 1 tablespoon butter
- ½ cup shredded Cheddar cheese
- 4 eggs

Instructions
1. Turn the oven to 400 degrees. Spread parchment paper over the surface of a large baking sheet.
2. After combining the butternut squash, chopped onion, Brussels sprouts, olive oil, one-half teaspoon of salt, and one-half teaspoon of black pepper in a large bowl, move the mixture to the baking sheet and toss to incorporate the ingredients.
3. Bake the vegetables for 20-22 minutes until they are soft and have a golden-brown color.
4. While the vegetables are roasting, melt the butter in a medium-sized saucepan set over medium heat.
5. To toast the oats, add them to the pan and heat for another 30 seconds. After adding the water, reduce the heat to maintain a simmer. When the oats have reached the desired consistency, which should be thick and chewy, reduce heat to low & continue simmering for another 8 to 10 minutes, adding additional water if required, mix in the shreds of cheese, then season with the remaining salt and ground black pepper. Keep warm.
6. Cook the eggs sunshine up or even over easy in a big skillet that has been oiled and is nonstick.
7. Put some oats in a bowl, layer it with some vegetables and an egg, and finish it off with some crumbled bacon.

Nutrition Facts
Calories: 460 calories, Protein: 19.9g, Carbs: 56.7g, Fat: 16.9g.

Farro Chicken Bowls

Prep Time: 20 /**Cook Time:** 20 /**Servings:** /**Difficulty level:** Moderate

Ingredients
For Bowl

- 1 cup tzatziki sauce
- Lemon wedges
- 2 cloves grated garlic
- Fresh dill & parsley, for garnish

- ½ cup feta crumbled cheese
- 2 tablespoons lemon juice
- ¼ teaspoon black pepper
- 1-pint halved cherry tomatoes
- 1 cup cooked Red Bob Mill Farro
- ½ teaspoon salt
- 1-pound boneless chicken skinless breasts
- 2 cups chopped cucumber
- ½ teaspoon kosher salt
- 1 cup sliced kalamata olives
- ½ red onion, sliced
- 1 tablespoon olive oil
- 3 tablespoons olive oil
- 1 teaspoon oregano dried
- Zest of 1 lemon
- 3 cups stock

For Tzatziki Sauce

- ¼ teaspoon dried dill
- 1 cup plain yogurt
- ½ teaspoon salt
- ½ teaspoon lemon juice
- 1 garlic clove
- 1 cucumber

Instructions

For Bowls

1. Farro must be rinsed and drained. Put the farro in a saucepan with enough salt and liquid, either water or stock, to cover it completely. Bring the whole shebang (everything) up to a boil, then instantly drop the heat to medium-low & let it simmer for half an hour. Remove any surplus water from the container.
2. For the sake of the chicken: Chicken breasts, lemon juice, olive oil, lemon zest, garlic, oregano, salt, & pepper should all be mixed in a zip bag that is a gallon in size. Marinate for at least four hours, preferably/overnight.
3. After heating the olive oil in a big pan over medium-high heat, place the chicken breasts in the skillet & cook for seven minutes before flipping them over and cooking for another five to seven minutes. The chicken is finished/done when the internal temperature reaches 165 degrees. Discard marinade.
4. Take the chicken/poultry out of the pan and rest for five minutes before slicing it.
5. To put together the Greek bowls, start by making a bed of farro in the bottom of the bowl or meal-prep container. Sliced chicken, tomatoes, cucumbers, olives, feta cheese, and tzatziki sauce should be placed on the pita before serving. Parsley and dill may be sprinkled on top, and the dish should be served with lemon wedges.

For Tzatziki Sauce

1. Prepare a big bowl by lining it with a fine-mesh sieve, then stuffing the sieve with a paper towel.
2. The cucumber & garlic clove should be grated using a cheese grater, and then they should be transferred to a filter to remove any extra moisture.
3. Combine the sliced/shredded cucumbers, garlic, yogurt, salt, lemon juice, and dill in a medium bowl. After giving everything a good stir to incorporate, put it in the refrigerator for an hour before serving.

Nutrition Facts
Calories: 585 calories, Protein: 35.9g,
Carbs: 45.5g, Fat: 30.4g.

Pumpkin-Peanut Butter Single-Serve Muffins

Prep time: 10 minutes/**Cook time:** 25 minutes/**Servings:** 2
Ingredients:
- 1 ½ cup canned pumpkin
- 2 tbsp powdered peanut butter
- 2 tbsp coconut flour
- 2 tbsp finely ground flaxseed
- ½ tsp baking powder
- 1 tbsp dried cranberries
- ½ cup water
- 2 large eggs
- ½ tsp vanilla extract
- olive oil cooking spray

Instruction:
1. Preheat the oven to 350°F.
2. In a medium bowl, stir together the powdered peanut butter, coconut flour,

flaxseed, baking powder, dried cranberries, and water.
3. In a separate medium bowl, whisk together the pumpkin and eggs until smooth.
4. Add the pumpkin mixture to the dry ingredients.
5. Stir to combine.
6. Add the vanilla. Mix together well.
7. Spray 2 (8-ounce) ramekins with cooking spray.
8. Spoon half of the batter into each ramekin.
9. Place the ramekins on a baking and carefully transfer the sheet to the preheated oven.
10. Bake for 25 minutes or until a toothpick in the center comes out clean.

Nutrition facts:
calories 219, fat 99g, protein 13g, carbs 24g, sugars 9g , fiber 10g , sodium 137mg

Breakfast Sausage Casserole

Prep time: 15 minutes/**Cook Time:** 3h 10 minutes /**Servings:** 6
Ingredients:
- 1 lb. pork sausage
- 1 tbsp garlic powder
- 1 tbsp dried thyme
- 1 tbsp rubbed sage
- ½ tbsp salt
- ½ cup green bell pepper
- ½ cup red bell pepper
- ½ cup red onion
- 1 tbsp ghee
- 12 eggs
- ½ cup coconut milk
- 1 tbsp nutritional yeast

Instruction:
1. Heat cast-iron pot for about 2 mins over medium heat then cut sausages into small pieces.
2. Add them to the pot to cook for 3 mins.
3. Add in garlic, thyme, sage, and salt to the pot and cook for 5 more mins.
4. Turn off the heat, stir in bell peppers and chopped onion.
5. Grease the slow cooker with ghee.
6. Pour the pork mixture into the bottom of your slow cooker.
7. In another large mixing bowl, mix eggs , milk and nutritional yeast until well combined.
8. Pour the egg mixture over the pork mixture then cover to cook 2-3hours or until the eggs are completely cooked.
9. Serve and enjoy when hot.

Nutrition facts:
calories 484, fat 38g, carbs 5g, proteins 29g, fiber 1.7g, sodium 129mg

Crustless Broccoli Cheese Quiche

Prep time: 5 minutes/**Cooking Time:** 2h 15 minutes/**Servings:** 8
Ingredients:
- 3 cups broccoli
- 9 eggs
- 1 tbsp olive oil
- ¾ tbsp salt and pepper
- ¼ powder onion
- 18 oz cream cheese
- 2 cups colby-jack cheese, shredded

Instruction:
1. Heat a large skillet with water over the stove to boil, add broccoli once the water starts to boil.
2. Cook for about 3 mins then drain and rinse it with cold water.
3. In a bowl add eggs, pepper , salt , onion powder and cheese.
4. Mix using a hand mixture until the cream cheese and eggs are well incorporated.
5. Grease the slow cooker with olive oil, add broccoli at the bottom then sprinkle over ½ cup of cheese.
6. Pour over the egg mixture on the broccoli.
7. Cover and cook on high for about 2 hours 15 mins.
8. Don't open the lid when cooking.

9. Sprinkle the remaining cheese and cover again for about 10 mins for cheese to melt.
10. Serve!

Nutrition facts:
Calories 297, fat 24g, carbs 4g, protein 16g, fiber 1g, potassium 246mg, sodium 552mg

Fruits Breakfast Salad

Prep time: 5 minutes/**Cooking Time**: 0 minutes/**Servings:**2
Ingredients:
- 1 cored and cubed pear
- ½ tsp cinnamon powder
- 1 peeled and sliced pear
- 2 oz toasted pepitas
- ½ lime juice

Instruction:
1. In a bowl, combine the pear using the pear, lime juice, cinnamon and pepitas, toss, divide between small plates and serve enjoying.

Nutrition facts:
calories 186, fat 4g, carbs 16g ,proteins 9g, fiber 3g, potassium 203mg, sodium 118mg

Pesto Egg Casserole

Prep time: 30 mins/**Cook Time:** 2 h 5 mins /**Servings:**8
Ingredients:
- 10 eggs, beaten
- 1 cup mozzarella, shredded
- 1 tbsp garlic, minced
- salt & pepper to taste
- 8-10 basil leaves, chopped
- 1 cup grape tomatoes, sliced and salted
- 8 oz mozzarella, fresh and cubed
- 6 oz pesto

Instruction:
1. Mix eggs, mozzarella cheese, minced garlic , salt , and pepper to taste in a mixing bowl.

2. Pour the mixture in a greased slow cooker.
3. Add basil, tomatoes, and mozzarella on top then cook on low for 2 hours.
4. Top with pesto, serve and enjoy.

Nutrition facts:
Calories 416, fat 36g, carbs 5g, protein 18g, fiber 1g, sodium 558mg , potassium 180mg

Kiwi Shake

Preparation time: 5 mins /**Cooking Time:** 0 mins /**Servings:**1
Ingredients:
- 2 cups kiwi cubed
- 1 pear, peeled and sliced
- 2 oranges, peeled and quartered
- 12-16 ice cubes, crushed

Ingredients:
1. Place kiwi, pear, oranges, and ice in a blender container.
2. Blend until smooth.
3. Pour into glasses and serve.

Nutrition Facts:
calories 139 , fat 15g , carbs 36g , protein 2g , fiber 1g , sodium 168mg , potassium 111mg

Greek Toast

Prep time:5 mins/**Cooking Time:** 0 mins /**Servings:**6
Ingredients:
- 1 ½ tsp. reduced-Fat: crumbled feta
- 3 sliced Greek olives
- ¼ mashed avocado
- 1 slice whole wheat bread
- 1 tbsp roasted red pepper hummus
- 1 sliced hardboiled egg
- 3 sliced cherry tomatoes

Instruction:
1. First , toast the bread and top it with ¼ mashed avocado and 1 tbsp hummus.
2. Add the cherry tomatoes, olives, hardboiled egg and feta.

Nutrition facts:

calories 333, fat 17g, carbs 33g, protein 16g, fiber 1g, sodium 296mg, potassium 125mg

Mushrooms Bites

Prep time: 5 mins/**Cooking Time:** 0 mins /**Servings:** 2

Ingredients:
- 4 Portobello mushroom caps
- 3 tbsp coconut aminos
- 2 tbsp sesame oil
- 1 tbsp fresh ginger, minced
- 1 small garlic clove, minced

Instruction:
1. Set your broiler to low, keeping the rack 6 inches from the heating source
2. Wash mushrooms under cold water and transfer them to a baking sheet
3. Take a bowl and mix in sesame oil, garlic, coconut aminos, ginger and pour the mixture over the mushroom tops
4. Cook for 10 mins

Nutrition facts:
Calories 196, fat 14g, carbs 14g, protein 7g, sg, fiber 1g, sodium 58mg, potassium 131mg

Whole-Grain Pancakes

Prep time: 5 minutes/**Cook time:** 10 minutes /**Servings:** 2

Ingredients:
- 2 teaspoons of sugar-free maple syrup
- 1 cup of whole-grain wheat flour
- 1/4 cup of skim milk
- 1 teaspoon of olive oil
- 1/2 teaspoon of baking powder

Instructions:
1. Combine baking powder & flour in a mixing bowl.
2. Combine the skim milk and olive oil.
3. Mix in all the ingredients till incorporated.
4. To make a pancake, preheat a nonstick skillet & spoon a small amount of batter onto the pan.
5. Cook for approximately 2 minutes on each side or till golden brown.
6. Sugar-free maple syrup can be drizzled over cooked pancakes.

Nutrition facts:
Calories 129, Total fat 2g, Protein 5g, Carbs 20g, Potassium 211mg, Sodium 10mg, Sugar 1g,

Omelet with Asparagus

Prep time: 10 minutes /**Cook time:** 10 minutes /**Servings:** 2

Ingredients:
- 3 oz. of chopped and boiled asparagus
- 3 beaten free-range eggs
- 2 tablespoons of low-fat milk
- 1 teaspoon of avocado oil
- 1/4 teaspoon of ground paprika
- 1/2 teaspoon of ground cumin
- A pinch of sea salt

Instructions:
1. Heat the avocado oil in a skillet.
2. In the meantime, mix the paprika & cumin powders together.
3. Add in eggs and milk.
4. In a hot skillet with the liquid, cook for around 2 minutes.
5. After that, cover the saucepan and add the chopped asparagus.
6. Cook the omelet for around 5 minutes on low flame.

Nutrition facts:
Calories 115, Total fat 7g, Protein 10g, Carbs 3g, Potassium 220mg, Sodium 101mg, Sugar 0.1g,

Breakfast Granola

Prep time: 10 minutes /**Cook time:** 20 minutes /**Servings:** 2

Ingredients:
- 2 tablespoons of cut oats
- 1/4 cup of chopped almonds
- 1 tablespoon of chia seeds
- 2 tablespoons of avocado oil
- 1 tablespoon of stevia
- 1 teaspoon of sesame seeds
- 1 teaspoon of sesame seeds

- 1/4 teaspoon of ground cinnamon
- Cooking spray

Instructions:
1. Heat the avocado oil with the stevia until it reaches a smooth consistency.
2. Toss in the sesame seeds, cinnamon powder, chia seeds, almonds, & oats after that.
3. Stir the ingredients till it is absolutely smooth.
4. After coating the baking pan with cooking spray, spread the almond mixture on it.
5. By flattening it, you can make a square out of it.
6. Preheat the oven to 345°F and bake the granola for around 20 minutes.
7. It should be portioned out once done.

Nutrition facts:
Calories 203, Total fat 11g, Protein 6g, Carbs 19g, Potassium 211mg, Sodium 21mg, Sugar 5g,

Breakfast Egg Toasts

Prep time: 10 minutes / **Cook time:** 10 minutes / **Servings:** 2
Ingredients:
- 3 whole-wheat bread slices
- 3 medium free-range eggs
- 1 teaspoon of olive oil
- 1/4 teaspoon of minced garlic
- A pinch of sea salt
- 1/4 teaspoon of ground black pepper

Instructions:
1. Heat the olive oil in a skillet.
2. After cracking the eggs, cook them for around 4 minutes.
3. In the meantime, rub the garlic cloves into the bread slices.
4. The bread is topped with scrambled eggs, a pinch of sea salt and freshly ground black pepper.

Nutrition facts:
Calories 157, Total fat 7g, Protein 9g, Carbs 13g, Potassium 182mg, Sodium 62mg, Sugar 1.5g,

Ricotta Toast with Pistachios and Honey

Prep time: 5 minutes / **Cook time:** 5 minutes / **Servings:** 2
Ingredients:
- 2 slices of multi-grain seeded bread
- 1/4 cup of part-skim ricotta cheese
- 2 tablespoons of chopped pistachios
- 1 teaspoon of sugar-free maple syrup

Instructions:
1. Toast the bread slices till they're lightly toasted and crunchy.
2. Spread the ricotta on the toast slices and evenly distribute the chopped nuts.
3. Drizzle with sugar-free maple syrup and serve.

Nutrition facts:
Calories 166, Total fat 7g, Protein 9g, Carbs 15g, Potassium 179mg, Sodium 130mg, Sugar 4g

Granny Smith Apples

Prep time: 0 mins / **Cook time:** 5 mins / **Serving:** 2
Ingredients:
- 3/4 cup unsweetened almond milk
- 1 cup rolled oats
- 1/2 c. raisins
- 1/4 teaspoon cinnamon powder
- 2 tablespoons date molasses or brown rice syrup

Instruction:
1. In a large mixing basin, mix the oats, almond milk, raisins, cinnamon, and date molasses (if using) and soak for 15 minutes.
2. When the cereal is ready to serve, grate the apple into it (or core and slice the apple separately before adding it to the cereal) and stir thoroughly.

Nutrition facts:
118 calories, 13 g fat, 12 g carbs, 7 g protein

Spiced Congee with Dates

Prep time: 0 mins /**Cook time:** 5 mins /**Serving:** 2
Ingredients:
- 4 cups brown rice, cooked
- 1/2 cup pitted and chopped dates
- 1/2 cup apricots, chopped
- 1 cinnamon stick, big
- 1/4 teaspoon cloves,
- ground season with salt to taste

Instruction:
1. In a large saucepan over moderate heat, bring 2 cups of water to a boil.
2. Include the Rice, apricots, dates, a cinnamon stick, and cloves Cook on a low Warm setting for 15 mins.
3. Season with salt and pepper.

Nutrition facts:
148 calories, 13 g fat, 16 g carbs, 22 g protein

Ham and Cheddar Omelets

Prep time: 2 mins /**Cook time:** 20 mins /**Serving:** 2
Ingredients:
- 2 steaks of ham
- 1 tablespoon of butter
- 1/2 onion (diced)
- 1 minced garlic clove
- 7 quail eggs
- 1 cup cheddar cheese, shredded
- 1/2 cup heavy cooker's cream
- Salt & pepper
- 1 tablespoon chopped chives

Instruction:
1. Preheat the oven to 400 degrees Fahrenheit.
2. Fry the ham steak and cube it.
3. Whisk together the eggs, heavy cream, salt, and pepper in a big mixing basin.
4. Whisk everything together until it's smooth.
5. Toss in the diced ham.
6. Melt the butter in an oven-safe pan.
7. 2 minutes of onion and garlic sautéing pour the egg/ham mixture into the pan.
8. Bake in the oven for 20 minutes, or until golden brown.
9. Finish with a sprinkling of minced chives.

Nutrition facts:
302 calories, 13 g fat, 14 g carbs, 20 g protein

Basic Oatmeal

Prep time: 0 mins /**Cook time:** 10 mins /**Serving:** 2
Ingredients:
- 1 cup oats, rolled
- 2 cups water or plant-based milk
- Season with salt to taste

Instruction:
1. In a small saucepan, bring the oats, plant-based milk, and salt to a boil.
2. Reduce to moderate-low Warm and simmer for 5 minutes, or until the oats are creamy.

Nutrition facts:
189 calories, 9 g fat, 12 g carbs, 24 g protein

Chorizo, Tomato & Grill Chili Frittata

Prep time: 0 mins /**Cook time:** 15 mins /**Difficulty Level:** Easy
Serving: 2
Ingredients:
- 6 oz. chorizo de carne
- 8 oz. green chili pepper (canned)
- 2/3 cup chopped/sliced red tomatoes
- Cheddar cheese, 2 oz.

Instruction:
1. In a big nonstick pan, brown the beef and pork chorizo for approximately 5 minutes over moderate high heat, breaking it up into bite-size pieces.
2. Remove and discard any surplus fat.
3. Prepare the broiler in the meanwhile.
4. Toss the chorizo in the pan with tomatoes, softly beaten eggs, cheese, and green chilies.

5. Cook for 5 minutes over high heat, then finish under the broiler for another 5 minutes, or until slightly puffed.
6. Serve right away.

Nutrition facts:
203 calories, 10 g fat, 16 g carbs, 24 g protein

Muesli with Coconut, Oats & Bananas

Prep time: 10 mins /**Cook time:** 10 mins /**Difficulty Level:** Easy /**Serving:** 2
Ingredients:
- 1 cup oats, rolled
- 3/4 cup almond milk, unsweetened
- 1/2 cup dates, pitted and chopped
- 1/4 cup roasted unsweetened coconut
- 1 peeled and sliced banana

Instruction:
1. In a mixing basin, mix all ingredients and soak for 15 minutes.

Nutrition facts:
228 calories, 12 g fat, 12 g carbs, 12 g protein

Steel-Cut Oats

Prep time: 0 mins /**Cook time:** 15 mins /**Difficulty Level:** Easy /**Serving:** 2
Ingredients:
- 1 cup oats, steel-cut
- 2 cups dried apple, chopped
- 1 cup pitted and chopped dates
- 1 stick of cinnamon

Instruction:
1. In a 2- or 4-quart slow cooker, mix the oats, dried apple, dates, cinnamon stick, and 4 cups water.
2. Cook for at least 8 hours, or until the oats are soft.
3. Before serving, take off the cinnamon stick.

Nutrition facts:
202 calories, 13 g fat, 12 g carbs, 24 g protein

Chapter 11: Lunch Recipes

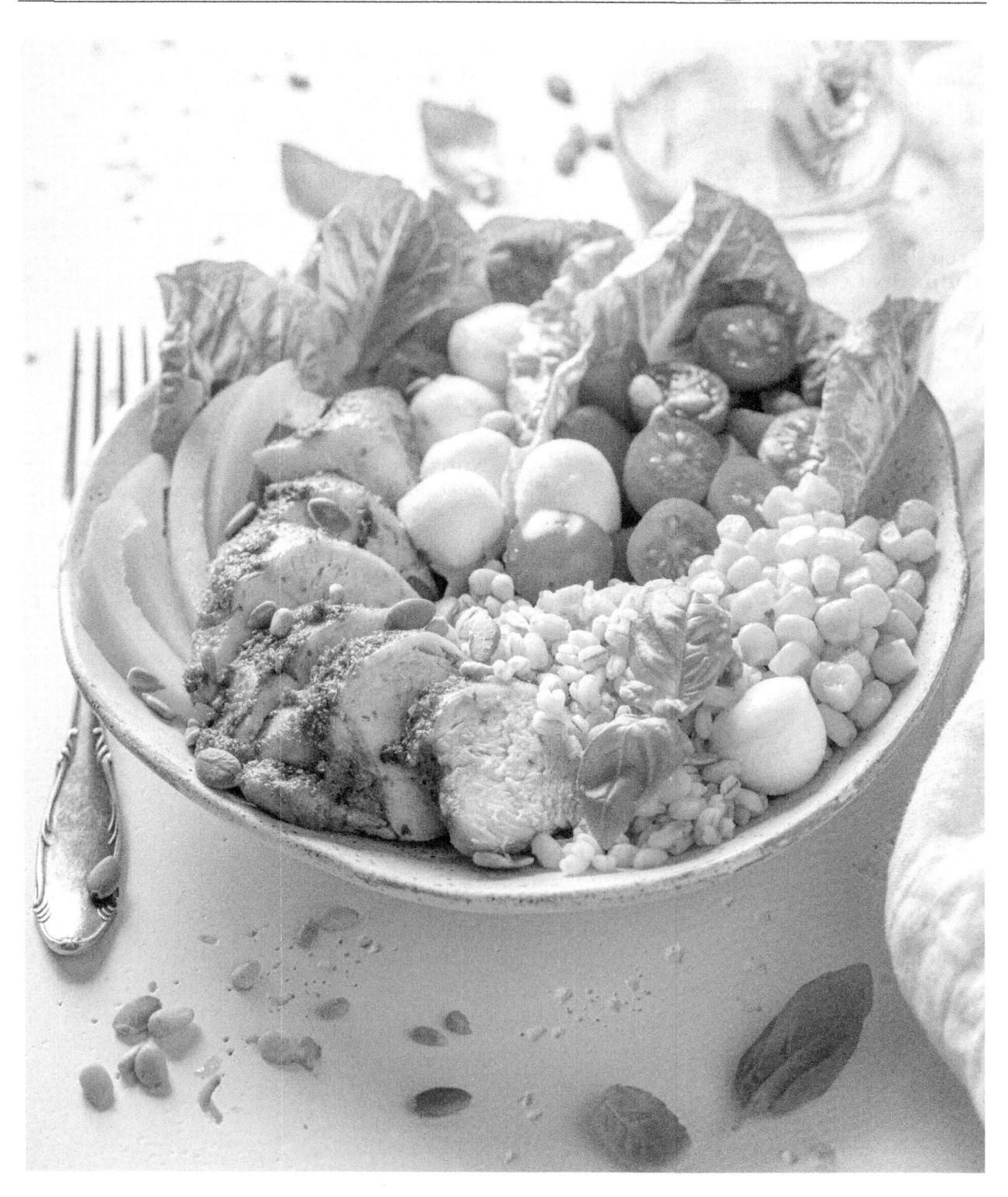

Pepper and Pesto Chicken Panini

Prep Time: 5 minutes/**Cook Time:** 2 minutes /**Servings:** 4/**Difficulty Level:** Easy

Ingredients

- Olive oil
- 1/2 cup red peppers
- 8 slices bread
- 3/4 pounds cooked chicken
- 4 oz fresh mozzarella, thinly sliced
- 4 Tbsp pesto

Instructions

1. Prepare a medium heat in a big cast-iron skillet or a grill pan that can be used on the stovetop.
2. Spread one spoonful of the pesto on each of the four slices of bread using the knife.
3. Place an equal quantity of sliced chicken, roasted red peppers, and mozzarella slices on each piece.
4. When the pan is heated, add a thin layer of olive oil, and fry the sandwiches two at a time, if required, till the bread is toasted and the cheese melt, which should take between three and four minutes on each side. If you want the greatest results, you should press the sandwiches down with a hefty pan.

Nutrition Facts
Calories: 445   calories, Protein: 38 g, Carbs: 32 g, Fat: 18g.

Caprese Sandwich

Prep Time: 10 minutes/**Cook Time:** 5 minutes /**Servings:** 4/**Difficulty Level:** Easy

Ingredients

- 2 large tomatoes
- Salt, add to taste
- 4 oz mozzarella
- 1 clove garlic
- black pepper to taste
- 1 baguette
- 1 Tbsp olive oil
- 15–20 fresh basil leaves
- 1 Tbsp balsamic vinegar

Instructions

1. Prepare the oven's broiler.
2. Toast the inside of the baguette by placing it under the broiler with the sliced sides facing up and keeping it at six inches from the heat for approximately two minutes.
3. To make fast garlic bread, just rub each half of the loaf with a clove of garlic cut in half. It will cause the essential oils in the garlic to be released by the crusty bread.
4. Assemble the sandwich starting with the bottom side of a baguette by alternating layers of tomato slices, mozzarella slices, and basil leaves.
5. Salt and plenty of freshly ground black pepper should be equally distributed throughout the dish.
6. To finish, garnish with a few drops of olive oil and lemon juice, and then place the other half of the baguette on top.
7. Divide the whole packet into quarters using a sharp knife.
8. Looking for a way to give your go-to sandwich a more exciting appearance? When you add a few of your favorite spreads or sauce to your caprese, it will taste like a completely different dish.

Nutrition Facts
Calories: 300 calories, Protein: 31 g, Carbs: 71 g, Fat: 17g

Feta Quiche

Prep Time: 10 minutes/**Cook Time:** 45 minutes /**Servings:** 6/**Difficulty Level:** Moderate

Ingredients

- pepper to taste
- 1/4 cup crumbled feta cheese
- 3 extra-large eggs
- 2 links cooked turkey
- 3/4 tsp kosher salt
- 2 Tbsp chopped tomatoes
- 1 frozen pie crust
- 1/2 can artichoke hearts
- 1 cup 2% milk

Instructions

1. Turn the oven up to 350 degrees Fahrenheit.
2. After beating the eggs until they are foamy, add the milk and the artichoke hearts, feta, tomato, sausage, and seasonings.
3. Pour into the bottom of the crust.
4. Put in the oven and cook for forty-five minutes until the eggs are fully set, a wooden skewer into the center will come out cleanly, and the top is softly golden brown. Place in the oven.
5. Probably wait 5 minutes for the cake to cool before slicing it and serving it.
6. They are already cooked inside various taste seasonings and ready to be diced up and used for scrambles, pasta, or stir-fries. Alternatively, they may be fried supplements containing onions and peppers to make an exceptional sandwich.

Nutrition Facts
Calories: 250 calories, Protein: 9.5 g, Carbs: 25 g, Fat: 14g

Asian Meatball

Prep Time: 15 minutes/**Cook Time:** 30 minutes /**Servings:** 4/**Difficulty Level:** Moderate

Ingredients

- 1 jalapeño pepper
- 1 tsp salt
- 1 Tbsp minced lemongrass
- 1 lb. ground chicken
- ginger scallion sauce
- 2 tsp sugar
- 1 small red onion
- pickled cucumber salad
- 2 cloves garlic
- Boston lettuce
- sriracha
- 1 Tbsp minced fresh ginger
- steamed rice
- 4–8 wooden skewers

Instructions

1. Warm-up a grill or grilling pan that has been cleaned and gently oiled.
2. In a large bowl, mix the ground beef with the onion, ginger, onion, lemongrass (if preferred), jalapeno, sugar, and salt. Using a gentle swirling motion, ensure that all ingredients are distributed equally throughout the mixture.
3. When the grill is ready, place the meatball skewers on it and cook them for about four to five minutes on each side, or until the exteriors of the meatballs have a light sear and the meatball are no longer pink on the inside. They should have a bouncy but firm texture to the touch when they are finished.
4. Utilize the lettuce and grains to form tiny wraps in the manner of Asian cuisine with the meatballs, decorating them with cucumbers and any sauces of your choosing.
5. Large lettuce leaves are often used in Korean cuisine as containers for grilled meats, grains, kimchi, and other sauces.
6. It might be anything: steak cooked on the barbecue, pork loin cooked on the grill, chicken portions cooked on the grill, or even vegetables cooked on the grill.
7. It's the same as eating a great burrito, but just a fifth of the calories. Feel free to be creative, but don't overlook the Sriracha sauce!

Nutrition Facts
Calories: 230 calories, Protein: 22 g, Carbs: 7 g, Fat: 12g

Avocado and Grilled Chicken

Prep Time: 15 minutes/**Cook Time:** 15 minutes /**Servings:** 4/**Difficulty Level:** Moderate

Ingredients

- ¼ cup dried cranberries
- 12 oz cooked chicken
- ¼ cup honey mustard vinaigrette
- ¼ cup goat cheese
- Salt, add to taste
- ¼ cup walnuts
- 1 avocado
- black pepper, add to taste
- 12 cups arugula

Instructions

1. Combine the chicken with the arugula, cranberry, avocado, cream cheese, walnuts, and vinaigrette in a large bowl. Season with salt and pepper to taste.
2. You may thoroughly include the dressing by either using your fingers or two forks.
3. Who doesn't enjoy a nice avocado? It is a superfood with many different nutrients in a single completely green serving.
4. Avocados are rich in several beneficial nutrients, including vitamin E, which is beneficial to both hair and skin; omega-3 fatty acids, which may help lower cholesterol levels; and folic acid, which is beneficial to pregnant women.

Nutrition Facts
Calories: 500 calories, Protein: 33 g, Carbs: 38 g, Fat: 24g

Fettuccine Alfredo Pasta

Prep Time: 15 minutes/**Cook Time:** 15 minutes /**Servings:** 4/**Difficulty Level:** Moderate

Ingredients
- 1 1/2 Tbsp butter
- 1/2 cup half and half
- 2 cloves garlic
- Salt to taste
- black pepper to taste
- 10 oz dried fettuccine
- 1 1/2 Tbsp flour
- 1/2 cup Parmesan
- 3/4 cup roasted red peppers
- 1 cup milk

Instructions

1. Start the cooking process by bringing a big pot of salted bring to a boil. After adding the pasta, cook it until it is firm to the bite, often 30 seconds to 1 minute shorter than recommended in the package directions.
2. Meanwhile, put butter in a pot of medium size and melt it over medium heat.
3. After incorporating the flour and continuing to cook for a further minute, the two ingredients should be completely combined. Whisking while gradually adding the milk and half-and-half should help avoid lumps from developing in the mixture.
4. To it, add the crushed red pepper and the garlic.
5. Reduce the heat to a low setting and let the mixture simmer for ten minutes.
6. The mixture should be puréed in a blender until it is very smooth, and the color should be consistent throughout.
7. After you have returned the mixture to the pan, whisk in the Parmesan.
8. After seasoning with salt and pepper, continue to boil the pasta until it has finished cooking.
9. After draining the pasta, put it in the pot it was cooking in.
10. To ensure an equal coating, toss.
11. Divide the mixture evenly between four heated dishes or plates.
12. Before inserting the pasta, stir 8 ounces of detached raw shrimp into the sauce for 2 minutes. Alternatively, stir 8 grams of leftover chicken into the sauce before adding the pasta.
13. After mixing the pasta with the sauce, add four cups of baby spinach and continue to simmer for about one minute, or until the spinach starts to wilt.
14. Before adding the pasta, stir in 2 cups worth of sautéed mushroom and roasted broccoli into the sauce.

Nutrition Facts
Calories: 390 calories, Protein: 23 g, Carbs: 68 g, Fat: 12g

Cheesesteak Sandwich

Prep Time: 15 minutes/**Cook Time:** 15 minutes /**Servings:** 4/**Difficulty Level:** Moderate

Ingredients
- 16 oz flank steak
- 1/4 cup blue cheese
- 2 tomatoes
- Salt to taste
- 4 sandwich rolls
- 2 cups arugula

- Caramelized onions
- 2 Tbsp olive-oil mayonnaise
- black pepper to taste
- 2 Tbsp Greek yogurt

Instructions

1. Mix the blue cheese, mayonnaise, and yogurt in a bowl. Set aside.
2. Heat the grill, stove grill pan, and cast-iron frying until hot.
3. To get medium-rare doneness, season the steak using pepper and salt, and then cook it for three to four minutes on each side. The steak is done when it is firm but will yield light pressure.
4. Probably wait 5 minutes until slicing the meat before allowing it to rest. Cut the meat into thin strips using a fork.
5. Arugula and tomatoes should be distributed evenly throughout the buns.
6. Add the steak and onions that have been caramelized to the top of each sandwich, and then sprinkle with blue cheese mayonnaise.
7. When you cut into a sirloin to check its doneness, you waste a significant amount of the meat's valuable liquids. Feel the food to determine if it is done.
8. When you press your finger against the middle of the steak, it should feel like a soft dish sponge when it is rare, like a firm but yielding Nerf football when it is medium, and like a hard but bouncy tennis ball when it is well done.
9. Regardless of how the meat feels to the touch, it is best to let it rest for five to ten minutes before cutting it. It allows the heated fluids to be reabsorbed by the flesh rather than your cutting board.

Nutrition Facts
Calories: 400 calories, Protein: 40 g, Carbs: 43 g, Fat: 14g

Meatball Soup

Prep Time: 10 minutes/**Cook Time:** 45 minutes /**Servings:** 4/**Difficulty Level:** Moderate

Ingredients

- 1 lb. ground beef
- ¼ cup bread crumbs
- 8 cups of low-sodium chicken stock
- 1 head escarole
- ½ Tbsp olive oil
- 2 medium eggs
- ½ cup finely grated Parmesan cheese
- Salt and ground black pepper to taste
- 1 onion
- 2 ribs celery
- ¾ cup small pasta
- 2 carrots

Instructions
In a mixing dish, combine the ground beef with the egg, bread crumbs, cheese, plus significant pinches of both salt and pepper.

1. Form the mixture into meatballs of about three-quarters of an inch in diameter, or slightly smaller than just a golf ball, taking care not to work overtime the ingredients.
2. Bring the olive oil to a simmer over medium-high heat in a large saucepan.
3. After adding the tomato, onions, and celery, continue to sauté the mixture for around 5 minutes, or until the veggies have become more tender.
4. After adding the stock and the escarole, reduce the heat to maintain a simmer in the soup.
5. Reduce the heat to a low setting, then add the meatball and spaghetti to the pan.
6. Continue to simmer for a further 8 - 10 mins, or until the meatball is fully cooked through it and the pasta has reached the desired al dente consistency.
7. Have a taste, and then season it to your liking with salt and black pepper.
8. To serve, sprinkle more cheese over the top of the soup.

Nutrition Facts
Calories: 333 calories, Protein: 11 g, Carbs: 12 g, Fat: 14g

Mashed Cauliflower

Preparation Time: 10 mins /**Cooking Time:** 10 mins /**Servings:** 4

Ingredients:
- ½ cup of cream cheese, whipped
- 1 head cauliflower, diced into florets
- 1 tsp seasoned salt or according to taste
- 2 cloves of minced garlic

Directions
1. Boil a large pot of water (lightly salted).
2. Cook the cauliflower in boiling water until it is tender; drain for about six minutes.
3. Dry the cauliflower to extract the moisture or liquid using a paper towel.
4. Blend cream cheese, cauliflower, seasoned salt, and garlic in a food processor till primarily smooth.

Nutritions facts:
102 calories | protein 4g | carbohydrates 9.4g | fat 6.4g | sodium 366.9mg

Bum's Lunch

Preparation Time: 15 mins /**Cooking Time:** 45 mins /**Servings:** 4

Ingredients:
- 4 potatoes, medium and thinly sliced
- 4 (4 oz) cube steaks
- 1 large, thinly sliced onion
- Salt and pepper according to taste
- 4 tsp margarine

Directions
1. Preheat the oven to 350°F
2. 4 squares of aluminum foil must be set down.
3. Place 1 cube of steak on each foil sheet.
4. Season the steaks with pepper and salt after spreading margarine over them.
5. Over each steak, place one sliced potato and a couple of onion rings.
6. If desired, season with pepper and salt once more.
7. Wrap the foil of all-around food and seal it to make a packet.
8. Placed on a baking pan.
9. In a preheated oven, bake for forty-five minutes until the beef is no pinker and the potatoes are soft.
10. Open with caution since it will emit hot steam.

Nutrition facts:
326 calories | protein 18.7g | carbohydrates 40.8g | fat 10g | sodium 90.1mg

High-Temp Pork Roast

Preparation Time: 15 mins/**Cooking Time:** 1 hr /**Servings:** 8

Ingredients:
- ¼ cup of Worcestershire sauce
- 2 lbs pork roast
- 2 tsp ground black pepper, coarse
- 1 tsp Montreal steak seasoning
- 1 tsp sea salt, coarse
- ½ tsp garlic powder
- 1 tsp onion powder

Directions
1. Preheat the oven to 500 degrees Fahrenheit.
2. To wet the outside of the roast, rinse it under cold running water.
3. Allow to air dry.
4. Spread Worcestershire sauce uniformly over the outside using a brush or paper towel.
5. On both sides, season the roast with salt, pepper, steak seasoning, garlic powder, and onion powder.
6. Place the roast fat-side up in a wide roasting pan on the center rack.
7. Roast for twenty minutes for medium, twenty-four minutes for medium-well, and twenty-eight minutes for well done in a preheated oven until done to your liking.
8. Switch off the oven and let the roast in for another forty minutes without opening the door.
9. Remove the pan from the oven and wrap it loosely with foil.
10. Enable a 10- to 15-minute rest period to allow the liquids to settle back into the roast.
11. Serve thinly sliced.

Nutrition facts:
105 calories | protein 13.2g | carbohydrates 2.5g | fat 4.4g | sodium 441.2mg

Chickpea Salad with Tomato and Red Onion

Preparation Time: 10 mins / **Cooking Time:** 2 hrs / **Servings:** 4

Ingredients:
- 2 tbsp chopped red onion
- 19 oz drained garbanzo beans
- 2 minced cloves of garlic
- ½ cup parsley, chopped
- 1 chopped tomato
- 1 tbsp lemon juice
- 3 tbsp olive oil
- Pepper and salt according to taste

Directions
1. Mix the red onion, chickpeas, garlic, parsley, tomato, olive oil, salt, pepper, and lemon juice in a big bowl.
2. Let it cool for two hours before serving.
3. Adjust the seasoning according to the taste.
4. Serve.

Nutrition facts:
262 calories | protein 7.3g | carbohydrates 33.3g | fat 11.8g | sodium 404.4mg

Chicken & Bacon Caesar Salad

Preparation Time: 10 mins / **Cooking Time:** 25 mins / **Servings:** 6

Ingredients
- 4 tablespoons olive oil
- 4 chicken breasts, skin on or off ½ ciabatta loaf, cubed
- 1 large cos (or Romaine) lettuce, leaves separated
- 75 g (3 oz) cooked crispy bacon rashers, broken into pieces
- 6 tablespoons Caesar salad dressing
- 25 g (1 oz) Parmesan cheese shavings
- Salt and pepper

Directions:
1. The water oven must be filled and preheated to 65 °C (149 °F).
2. In a big, heavy-based frying pan, heat 2 tablespoons of oil.
3. Season the chicken breasts with salt and pepper and sear over medium-high heat for 1–2 minutes on each side until golden.
4. Remove from the pan, cool slightly, then divide a single layer between 2 small cooking pouches.
5. Vacuum seal at the sealer's natural/dry setting and submerge for 1 hour.
6. Meanwhile, put the ciabatta cubes on a foil-lined grill pan and drizzle over the remaining olive oil.
7. Toast for about 5 minutes under a preheated medium grill, turning periodically until golden and crisp.
8. Withdraw and set aside.
9. Remove from their pouches the chicken breasts, pat dry with kitchen paper, and slice into bite-sized bits.
10. Tear the lettuce leaves roughly and put them with the chicken and most bacon bits in a salad bowl.
11. Apply the salad dressing and toasted bread cubes and toss well to match.
12. Sprinkle and serve immediately over the reserved bacon bits and the Parmesan shavings.

Nutrition facts:
391 calories | proteins 15g | carbohydrates 3.6g | fat 35.2g | sodium 725.2mg

Barbecued Poussins with Chili Corn Salsa

Preparation Time: 10 mins / **Cooking Time:** 45 mins / **Servings:** 4

Ingredients
- finely grated rind and juice of 1 lime
- 2 tbsp Cajun spice mix
- 3 tbsp olive oil
- 2 poussins, each jointed in half and flattened slightly, 5 cm (2 inches) thick
- 175 g (6 oz) can of sweetcorn

- 1 red chili, finely chopped
- ¼ cucumber, finely chopped
- Salt and pepper

Directions
1. The water oven must be filled and preheated to 65 °C (149 °F).
2. The turkey fillets are seasoned with salt and pepper and divided into 2 small cooking pouches.
3. Vacuum seal in the sealer's natural/dry environment and submerge for 1½ hours.
4. Meanwhile, heat the oil in a big, heavy-based frying pan over medium heat and cook the garlic for a few seconds.
5. Passata, sugar, and oregano are added. Simmer until thick and pulpy for 5-8 minutes. Then, if the frying pan is not ovenproof, pour it into a small, ovenproof gratin dish.
6. Take the turkey fillets from their pouches and place them in the tomato sauce.
7. Mix half of the Parmesan with the breadcrumbs, then scatter over the turkey fillets.
8. Once the cheese has melted and the sauce is bubbling, scatter over the mozzarella and remaining Parmesan and position under a preheated grill for 2-3 minutes.
9. If needed, serve with crusty bread.

Nutritions facts:
334 calories | protein 23.3g | carbohydrates 21.4g | fat 17g | sodium 1020mg

Kale Lasagna with Meat Sauce

Preparation Time: 10 minutes / **Cooking Time:** 15 minutes / **Servings:** 1
Ingredients:
- 1 pound Italian pork sausage, casings removed
- 1 pound of ground beef
- ½ cup minced onion
- Two cloves of garlic, crushed
- 1 (14.5 ounces) can of crushed tomatoes
- 2 (6 ounces) cans of tomato paste
- ½ cup vegetable broth
- Two tablespoons of Italian seasoning
- salt and ground black pepper to taste
- 1 (16 ounces) package of lasagna noodles
- 1 (16 ounces) container of ricotta cheese
- 2 cups chopped kale
- One egg
- 1 cup grated Parmesan cheese
- 1-pound shredded mozzarella cheese

Directions:
1. Preheat the oven carefully to 375° F.
2. In a large saucepan over medium-high heat, brown and stir Italian sausage, ground beef, onion, and garlic until meats are browned and crumbly, 5 to 7 minutes.
3. Crush the tomatoes, and add the tomato paste, vegetable broth, Italian spice, salt, and pepper to taste.
4. Bring to a low boil. Reduce the heat to low and cook, stirring periodically, for about 1 hour.
5. Meanwhile, heat a big pot of gently salted water.
6. Cook the lasagna noodles in boiling water for 8 minutes, tossing periodically, until soft yet firm to the biting.
7. Combine the ricotta cheese, kale, and egg in a mixing dish.
8. Layer the lasagna in a 9x13-inch baking dish, beginning with a small amount of meat sauce and noodles, then 1/2 of the ricotta mixture, more noodles, then the majority of the remaining meat sauce.
9. Continue with the remaining Parmesan cheese, 1/2 of the mozzarella cheese, noodles, remaining ricotta mixture, and meat sauce.
10. Finish with the remaining mozzarella cheese.
11. 30 to 45 minutes bake uncovered in a warm oven until bubbling and golden.
12. Allow 10 minutes to cool and solidify before cutting.

Nutritions facts:
310 calories | protein 23.7g | carbohydrates 20.4g | fat 17g | sodium 910 mg

Blue Cheese, Spinach Meat Loaf Muffins

Preparation Time: 10 minutes /**Cooking Time:** 15 minutes /**Servings:** 1

Ingredients:
- 1 ½ pounds lean ground beef
- ¾ cup crumbled blue cheese
- ½ cup diced onion
- ½ cup Italian bread crumbs
- ½ cup chopped fresh spinach
- Two eggs
- Two tablespoons of Worcestershire sauce

Directions:
1. Preheat the oven carefully to 375°F (190 degrees C).
2. Cooking spray should be sprayed into a large muffin tin.
3. In a large mixing bowl, combine ground beef, blue cheese, onion, bread crumbs, spinach, eggs, and Worcestershire sauce until thoroughly combined.
4. Divide the meat mixture equally among the prepared muffin cups.
5. Thirty minutes in a preheated oven until the middle is no longer pink.
6. In the middle, an instant-read thermometer should read at least 160 degrees F.

Nutritions facts:
315 calories | protein 22.3g | carbohydrates 18.4g | fat 17g | sodium 850mg

Syrian Rice with Meat

Preparation Time: 10 minutes /**Cooking Time:** 15 minutes /**Servings:** 1

Ingredients:
- ¼ cup butter
- 2 pounds of ground beef
- Two teaspoons salt
- ½ teaspoon ground allspice
- ½ teaspoon ground cinnamon
- ½ teaspoon ground black pepper
- 4 ½ cups chicken broth
- 2 cups long-grain white rice
- Two tablespoons butter
- ½ cup pine nuts

Directions:
1. In a large saucepan over medium-high heat, melt 1/4 cup butter.
2. Mix in the ground meat, salt, allspice, cinnamon, and black pepper—Cook for 7 to 10 minutes, or until the meat is browned.
3. Pour in the chicken broth and rice.
4. Bring to a boil, covered.
5. Cook until the liquid has been absorbed, about 20 minutes.
6. Meanwhile, melt two tablespoons of butter in a small pan over medium heat.
7. Cook until the pine nuts are gently toasted, 3 to 5 minutes.
8. Before serving, toss pine nuts into the rice and meat combination.

Nutritions facts:
334 calories | protein 23.3g | carbohydrates 21.4g | fat 17g | sodium 1020mg

Deer Meat

Preparation Time: 10 minutes /**Cooking Time:** 15 minutes /**Servings:** 1

Ingredients:
- 1 ½ pounds venison (deer meat)
- Two onions, chopped
- 4 cups fresh mushrooms, sliced
- Three tablespoons butter
- One clove of garlic, minced
- 1 (6 ounces) can of tomato paste
- One teaspoon of all-purpose flour
- 1 cup sour cream
- One teaspoon salt
- One pinch of mustard powder
- ⅛ teaspoon dried parsley

Directions:
1. In a large pan over medium heat, melt butter or margarine.
2. Sauté the onions till transparent, then add the meat and brown it.

3. After gently browning the meat, add mushrooms, garlic, tomato paste, flour, sour cream, salt, mustard powder, and parsley.
4. Stir everything together, then decrease the heat to low and let it simmer for 20 to 30 minutes.
5. The longer it cooks, the softer the flesh becomes.
6. Enjoy!

Nutritions facts:
301 calories | protein 18.3g | carbohydrates 15.4g | fat 17g | sodium 920mg

Sicilian Meat Roll

Preparation Time: 10 minutes /**Cooking Time:** 15 minutes /**Servings:** 1
Ingredients:
- Two eggs, beaten
- ½ cup tomato juice
- ¾ cup soft bread crumbs
- Two tablespoons of snipped fresh parsley
- ½ teaspoon dried oregano, crushed
- ¼ teaspoon sea salt
- ¼ teaspoon ground black pepper
- One clove of garlic, minced
- 2 pounds lean ground beef
- 1 (6 ounces) package of thinly sliced ham
- 1 (6 ounces) package of shredded mozzarella cheese

Directions:
1. Combine the eggs and tomato juice in a large mixing basin.
2. Combine the bread crumbs, parsley, oregano, salt, pepper, garlic, and ground beef in a mixing bowl.
3. Thoroughly combine—Preheat the oven carefully to 350°F (175 degrees C).
4. Pat and shape the meat into a 10x8 inch rectangle on a piece of foil or waxed paper.
5. Place ham slices on the meat, leaving a border around the edges.
6. Tear up the cheese pieces, leaving one whole, and scatter over the ham.
7. Gently wrap up the meat, lifting with foil or waxed paper starting from the short end.
8. Seal the meat's edges and ends.
9. Place the roll in a 9x13 inch baking dish, seam side down.
10. Bake for 75 minutes in a preheated oven.
11. Cut the reserved cheese slice into four triangles.
12. Place the triangles on top of the bread— Bake for 2 minutes, or until the cheese melts.

Nutritions facts:
335 calories | protein 23.4g | carbohydrates 21.5g | fat 17g | sodium 1010mg

Chicken-Apricot Casserole

Preparation time: 10 minutes /**Cooking Time:** 55 minutes /**Servings:** 4
Ingredients:
- 2 chopped garlic cloves,
- 1 sliced onion,
- 2 teaspoons of ground cumin
- 8 chicken thighs,
- 1 1/4 cup of chicken broth
- 2 tsp of ground coriander
- 5 pitted and quartered apricots,
- 2 tbsp of canola oil
- 3 carrots, halved crosswise,
- 6 to 8 thick fingers,
- Chopped fennel leaves.
- Salt and pepper to taste.

Direction:
1. Fennel should be split lengthwise and cut crosswise into slices on a cutting board.
2. In a large pan, heat the oil and cook the chicken thighs, flipping periodically, until golden brown on both sides, for about 5 to 10 minutes.
3. Remove it from the pan.
4. Sauté the garlic and onion in the pan for approximately 5 minutes, or until tender and golden.
5. Add all the spices and cook for 1 minute before adding the stock.
6. Return the chicken and the fennel and carrots to the pan.

7. Bring the water to a boil.
8. Stir thoroughly, then cover and cook for 30 minutes, or until the chicken is cooked.
9. Take off the cover.
10. If there is too much liquid, decrease it somewhat by boiling.
11. Stir the apricots into the casserole gently to blend.
12. Cook for another 5 minutes over low heat.
13. Season with salt and pepper to taste.
14. Serve with a sprinkling of fennel leaves.

Nutritional facts:
calories: 280 kcal, protein: 26 g, carbohydrates: 18 g, Fat: 13 g, Cholesterol: 49.5 mg, Fiber: 0.7 g

Pasta with grilled chicken, white beans, and mushrooms

Preparation time: 10 minutes /**Cooking Time:** 20 minutes /**Servings:** 6
Ingredients:
- 1/2 cup of chopped white onion.
- 1 tablespoon of olive oil
- 1 cup of white beans, cooked or canned (no salt added)
- 2 skinless, boneless chicken breasts,
- 4 ounces each
- 1 cup of sliced mushrooms
- 1/4 cup of chopped fresh basil.
- 2 tablespoons of chopped garlic
- 12 ounces of uncooked roselle pasta
- black pepper: ground, to taste
- 1/4 cup of grated Parmesan cheese

Direction:
1. In a charcoal grill, create a fire, or heat a broiler or gas grill.
2. Spray the broiler pan or grill rack gently with cooking spray spaced 4 to 6 inches away from the heat source.
3. For 5 minutes, grill or broil each side of the chicken until it turns brown and is cooked.
4. Allow 5 minutes for the chicken to rest on a chopping board before slicing into strips.
5. Heat the olive oil in a large nonstick frying pan over medium heat.
6. Sauté the mushrooms and onions for approximately 5 minutes, or until they are soft.
7. Combine the basil, garlic, white beans, and grilled chicken pieces in a large mixing bowl.
8. Keep it warm.
9. Bring a big saucepan 3/4 full of water to a boil.
10. Add and cook pasta for 10 to 12 minutes, or according to package instructions, until the pasta is al dente (tender).
11. Drain all of the water from the pasta.
12. Add the mixture of chicken to the pasta in the saucepan.
13. Toss to distribute the ingredients properly.
14. Distribute the spaghetti amongst the plates.
15. Garnish with 1 tablespoon of Parmesan cheese and black pepper on top of each.
16. Serve right away.

Nutritional facts:
Calories: 341 kcal, protein: 21 g, carbohydrates: 53 g, Fat: 5 g, Cholesterol: 30 mg, Fiber: 4 g

Lemon Rosemary Chicken

Preparation time: 10 minutes /**Cooking Time:** 60 minutes /**Servings:** 8
Ingredients:
- 1 whole chicken, 3 to 4 pounds (1.4 to 1.8 kg)
- 1/2 cup lemon juice
- 1 teaspoon dried rosemary

Direction:
1. Split chicken in half, cutting along backbone and breastbone.
2. Place in a resealable plastic bag with lemon juice and rosemary.

3. Marinate for at least two hours, turning frequently.
4. Preheat the grill, making one side hot and the other low heat.
5. Cook over the low side with grill covered, turning several times, for about 1 hour or until done.
6. Discard the skin.

Nutritional facts:
Calories: 33 kcal, protein: 5 g, carbohydrates: 1 g, Fat: 1 g, Cholesterol: 17 mg, Fiber: 0 g

Chicken Zucchini Pie

Preparation time: 5 minutes / **Cooking Time:** 40 minutes / **Servings:** 6

Ingredients:
- 1 cup cooked chicken breast, cubed
- 1 cup zucchini, cubed
- 1 cup tomatoes, chopped
- 1 cup onion, chopped
- 1/4 cup Parmesan cheese, shredded
- 1 cup skim milk
- 1/2 cup Reduced-Fat Biscuit Mix
- 1/2 cup egg substitute
- 1/4 teaspoon black pepper

Direction:
1. Preheat the oven to 400°F and coat a 9-inch (23-cm) pie plate with nonstick vegetable oil spray.
2. Mix chicken, zucchini, tomatoes, onion, and cheese and spoon evenly into the prepared pie plate.
3. Beat remaining ingredients in a blender or with a wire whisk until smooth.
4. Pour evenly over the chicken mixture.
5. Bake for 35 minutes until a knife inserted in the center comes out clean.
6. Let stand 5 minutes before cutting.

Nutritional facts:
Calories: 156 kcal, protein: 15 g, carbohydrates: 15 g, Fat: 4 g, Cholesterol: 25 mg, Fiber: 1 g

Chicken Etouffee

Preparation time: 10 minutes / **Cooking Time:** 25 minutes / **Servings:** 4

Ingredients:
- 2 tablespoons unsalted margarine
- 1 cup onion, chopped
- 1 tablespoon flour
- 1-pound boneless chicken breasts
- 3/4 cup water
- 2 tablespoons lemon juice
- 2 tablespoons no-salt-added tomato paste
- 1/4 teaspoon cayenne pepper
- 2 tablespoons scallions, sliced
- 1 tablespoon dried parsley

Direction:
1. In a saucepan with a tight-fitting lid, melt margarine, add onion, and cook over medium heat until tender.
2. Stir in the flour, and blend well.
3. Add chicken, water, lemon, tomato paste, and cayenne pepper.
4. Cook over low heat for 15 minutes, adding more water if necessary.
5. Add scallions and parsley.
6. Serve over steamed rice.

Nutritional facts: Calories: 208 kcal, protein: 27 g, carbohydrates: 8 g, Fat: 7 g, Cholesterol: 66 mg, Fiber: 1 g

Tasty Fish Fillets

Prep time: 10 mins / **Cook time:** 10 mins / **Serving:** 3

Ingredients:
- 4 fillets (medium size) of tilapia fish
- 3 cloves garlic chopped
- ½ cup Parmesan cheese
- 2 tbsp chopped parsley
- 2 tbsp freshly squeezed lemon juice
- 2 tbsp olive oil
- ½ tsp cayenne pepper
- ½ tsp pepper
- Low salt to taste

Direction:
1. First, preheat the grill at a medium heat setting.
2. Wash the fish fillets' water and dry with a paper towel.
3. Put all the fish fillets in the baking dish.

4. Mix garlic, cayenne pepper, salt, olive oil, black pepper, and lemon juice in a bowl.
5. Pour this over the fish fillets.
6. Now grill the fish fillets on the grill.
7. Fish usually takes less time to grill.
8. Grain each side for 3 to 4 minutes, then take off from the grill into a serving platter.
9. Top the fish fillets with parmesan cheese and fresh parsley.
10. Serve hot with fresh lemon slices.

Nutritional facts: Calories: 422 kcal Carbohydrates: 21 g Protein: 22 g Fats: 30 g Sodium: 500 mg

Grilled Dory Fish

Preparation Time: 15 minutes /**Cooking Time:** 1 hour /**Serving:** 3
Ingredients:
- 4 fillets of dory
- 1 tsp onion Powder
- ½ cup salt
- ½ tsp black pepper
- 1 tsp ginger powder
- 1 tsp garlic powder
- Coriander for garnish
- Lemon slices for garnish

Direction:
1. Wash the fish fillets with cold running water.
2. Next, prepare a rub by mixing all the ingredients and spices.
3. Apply the rub on the fish fillets generously.
4. Wrap the fish fillets in cling film and refrigerate them overnight.
5. The next day, the fish fillets are brought to room temperature.
6. Prepare the electric Smoker with wood chips and water.
7. Turn it on at 220°F.
8. When the fillets are at room temperature, wash them and pat them dry.
9. Preheat the grill.
10. Grill the fish fillets for 4 minutes on each side.
11. Let the fillets rest for 30 minutes before serving.
12. Garnish the fish fillets with coriander and lemon slices for serving.

Nutritional facts:
Calories: 287 kcal Carbohydrates: 22g Protein: 18 g Fats: 14 g Sodium: 541 mg

Tuna and Broccoli Pasta

Prep time: 45 minutes /**Cooking time:** 30 times /**Serving:** 6
Ingredients:
- 400g tuna fish fillets
- 500g macaroni
- 250g broccoli chopped
- 2 tablespoon flour
- 3 slices of sourdough bread
- 500ml milk
- 2 red onions, finely chopped
- 4 tablespoon vinegar
- 50g butter
- 2 tablespoon mustard
- 250g cheddar cheese
- 2 tablespoon capers
- 3 tablespoon chopped parsley

Direction:
1. Heat the grill at a medium heat level.
2. Wash the tuna fillets and rub some olive oil on them.
3. Season with salt and freshly ground pepper.
4. Grain the tuna on each side for 4 to 7 minutes.
5. Take care that the fish is not burnt.
6. Set aside on a cutting board.
7. Cut into thick slices and set aside.
8. Meanwhile, preheat the oven to 300°F.
9. Mix onion and vinegar in a small bowl.
10. Set aside.
11. Cook pasta for 8 minutes in boiling water.
12. Drain the water and put the pasta aside.
13. Put broccoli in a steamer and steam for five minutes.
14. Prepare the white sauce.
15. Take a saucepan, and melt some butter.
16. Add some flour slowly and mix.

17. No lumps should be formed.
18. Cook for at least two minutes.
19. Turn off the heat and add milk gradually and mix well.
20. Take care that no lumps are formed.
21. Turn on the heat and cook on a high flame for two minutes.
22. Turn off the heat, add the mustard and cheese, and mix until the cheese melts.
23. Add the pasta, broccoli, and half of the parsley to this sauce.
24. Drain the vinegar from the onion and add the onion to the white sauce.
25. Put all of this in a large oven-safe dish.
26. Scatter some sourdough pieces on the top of the dish.
27. Bake for 30 minutes.
28. The dish will be bubbly after taking out of the oven.
29. Wait for it to stop bubbling.
30. Serve the pasta with grilled tuna on the side.
31. Serve immediately

Nutritional facts:
Calories: 340 kcal Carbohydrates: 36 g Protein: 26 g Fats: 10 g Sodium: 121 mg

Chicken with Herbs

Preparation Time: 10 mins /**Cooking Time:** 20 mins /**Serving:** 3
Ingredients:

- 2.5 kg chicken wings
- ½ cup olive oil
- 2 garlic minced.
- 2 tbsp rosemary leaves
- 2 tbsp fresh basil leaves
- 2 tbsp lemon juice
- 1 ½ tsp potassium salt
- 1 tsp pepper
- 2 tbsp oregano

Direction:
1. Prepare the chicken wings by trimming them.
2. Wash the wings under cold running water.
3. You can break the wings into half or use them as it is.
4. Add all ingredients and herbs to a large mixing bowl and make a smooth mixture.
5. Save half and toss the chicken wings in the other half.
6. Use your hands to toss the wings in the mixture, so it is evenly applied.
7. Preheat the grill.
8. Arrange the chicken wings on the grill.
9. Grill for 7 minutes on each side.
10. Check for doneness.
11. The meat on the wings should be tender.
12. Take off the wings from the grill.
13. Let them rest for 5 to 10 minutes before serving.

Nutritional facts:
Calories: 472 kcal Carbohydrates: 5.2 g Protein: 25 g Fats: 40g Sodium: 74 mg

Chapter 12: Dinner Recipe

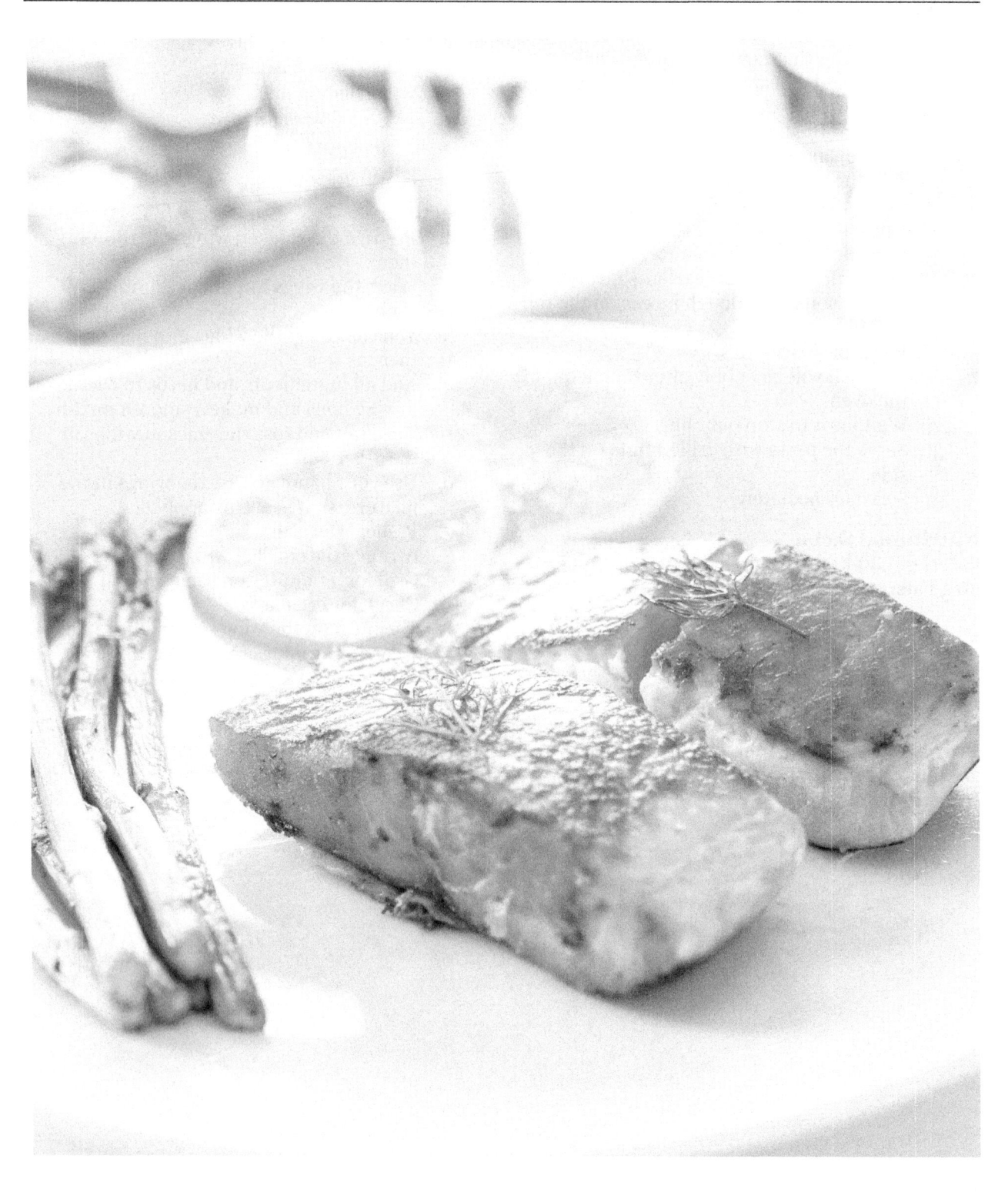

Sweetened Potato Curry with Chickpeas

Prep Time: 30 minutes/**Cook Time:** 20 /**Servings:** 6/**Difficulty level:** Moderate

Ingredients

- Cinnamon - 2 teaspoon
- Basmati rice or brown rice, for serving
- Chickpeas, rinsed and drained - 1 can
- Chopped fresh cilantro for garnish - ¼ cup
- Diced tomatoes, can substitute fresh if available - 1 ounce
- Sweet onions, chopped - ½ large
- Scallions – 2 thinly sliced
- Potatoes- 2 large sweet, peeled and diced
- Cumin - 1 tablespoon
- Curry powder - 2 tablespoons
- Canola oil - 1 -2 teaspoon
- Spinach - 10 ounces fresh, washed, stemmed, and coarsely chopped
- Cinnamon - 1 teaspoon
- Water - ½ cup

Instructions

1. The first step is to chop all the vegetables. You can chop all your vegetables, small or large, depending on your preference. You may opt to prepare the sweet potatoes in any way you wish.
2. Some people prefer to peel, cut, and cook vegetables in a vegetable steamer. Do this for approximately 15 minutes.
3. In this step, Baking & boiling work nicely too.
4. While sweet potatoes cook, boil 1-2 tablespoons of vegetable oil on moderate flame.
5. Add some onions and cook for 2-3 minutes, or till they begin chili soften.
6. Then, add your curry powder, cumin, and cinnamon, and mix to cover the onions equally with spices.
7. In this step, add tomatoes and their juices and chickpeas, and mix to incorporate them.
8. Add 1 by 2 cups water and bring heat up to a hard simmer for approximately a minute or two.
9. Following, add chopped fresh spinach, a few handfuls at the moment, stirring to coat in cooking liquid.
10. Once all the greens are put in the pan, continue cooking until just soft, about 3 minutes.
11. Add the cooked potatoes to the broth, and swirl to coat.
12. In this step, cook for another 3 to 5 minutes, or till flavors are well blended.
13. Add to a serving dish, mix with fresh cilantro, then serve hot.
14. This meal is wonderful, served over basmati as well as brown rice.
15. Your dish is ready to be served. For drink, have it with water because any soda might be harmful and ruin your intermittent fasting.

Nutrition Facts

Calories: 160 calories, Proteins: 56 g, Carbs: 55 g, Fat: 20 g

Black Eyed Crock Pot Peas

Prep Time: 45 minutes/**Cook Time:** 10 hours and 5 minutes/**Servings:** 6/**Difficulty level:** Moderate

Ingredients

- Cinnamon - 2 teaspoon
- Celery – 1 stalk, chopped
- Black-eyed peas - 2 cans bag dried
- Chicken broth - 2 cans
- Tomatoes - 1 can be diced with green chilies
- Del Monte zesty jalapeno pepper - 1can
- Ham hock - 1 small sized

Instructions

1. This recipe only consists of two steps. The first step is to prepare the black-eyed peas.
2. Soak the black-eyed peas in water for the time recommended on the package.
3. Bring together all the ingredients listed above in a pot.
4. Then, simmer on low flame for about 9 to 10 hours after combining all the ingredients.

Nutrition Facts

Calories: 200 calories, Proteins: 90 g, Carbs: 89 g, Fat: 13 g

Chicken Sheet Pan Brussel Sprouts

Prep Time: 40 minutes/**Cook Time:** 35 minutes/**Servings:** 4/**Difficulty level:** Moderate

Ingredients

- Herbs de Provence – 1 teaspoon
- Olive oil – 3 tablespoons
- chicken thighs – 4 skins
- Carrots – 4 cuts on the bias
- Brussels sprouts – 1 by 2 cups, halved

Instructions

1. The initial step in this yummy recipe is to set the temperature in the oven to 400 degrees Fahrenheit.
2. After that, Place the sliced veggies in a bowl.
3. Now that all the veggies are in a bowl, add 1 and a half tablespoons of olive oil with 1 by 2 teaspoons of herbs, salt, and pepper to taste.
4. Sprinkle all over vegetables thoroughly.
5. Now comes the next step, Spread the vegetables out on a baking sheet.
6. Place the chicken thighs in the same bowl as the marinade. You should also sprinkle this with salt and pepper, one and a half tablespoons of olive oil, and half a teaspoon of herbs.
7. Make sure that the chicken is covered in a rub.
8. Now what you must do is arrange the chicken in the pan.
9. Place chicken in oven and roast for approximately 30 to 35 minutes, or until it is cooked thoroughly.
10. Approaching the last few steps, you should heat the oven to broil and cook for one or two minutes if you want the skin on your chicken or vegetables to get a little crisper. Put up an eye on it in case it catches fire.
11. You can also squeeze some lemon juice for that extra tangy flavor.

Nutrition Facts
Calories: 220 calories, Proteins: 60 g, Carbs: 49 g, Fat: 25 g

Cauliflower Thin Crust Pizza

Cook Time: 40 minutes/**Servings:** 4/**Difficulty level:** Moderate

Ingredients

- Egg - 1 beaten
- Salt – 1 pinch
- Soft cheese – 1 cup
- Oregano – 1 teaspoon
- Cauliflower – 1 Medium-sized

Instructions

1. The first step is to prepare the oven to 400 degrees Fahrenheit.
2. To prepare cauliflower rice, you will need to pulse groups of fresh cauliflower florets inside a food processor until the cauliflower reaches a consistency like rice.
3. Put about a centimeter and a half of water into a large pot, then bring it to a boil. After adding the "rice," cover the pot and let it simmer for around four to five minutes. Drain through a strainer with a fine mesh.
4. After you have strained the rice, place it on a fresh dishtowel that is rather thin. Wrap the rice that has been steamed in the dishtowel, wrap it up, and then squeeze all the extra liquid out of the rice!
5. It is incredible how much additional liquid will be produced, resulting in a lovely and dry crust once it has been baked.
6. The next thing is to combine the cooked rice that has been drained, the beaten egg, the goat cheese, and the seasonings in a large bowl.
7. Do not be afraid to make use of the tools at your disposal. You want everything to be thoroughly combined.) It won't be like any pizza bread you've ever dealt with, but you don't need to worry about falling apart because it will still be edible.
8. In this step, you will have to apply some pressure to the dough and spread it out on a baking sheet of paper that has been prepared with parchment paper.
9. It must be lined with parchment paper to prevent it from sticking.

10. Maintain a thickness of about 3 by 8 inches for the dough, and if you want a "crust" impression, make the sides slightly higher than the center.
11. Cook for 35 to 40 minutes at 400°F. When the crust is done, it should be firm and have a golden-brown color.
12. Now is the moment where you must add all your preferred toppings, including sauce, cheese, or any toppings that you might enjoy.
13. Rest the pizza back on the stove at 400 degrees Fahrenheit and continue baking for another 5 to 10 minutes until all cheese is melted and bubbling.
14. The last step has finally come. Now slice, serve as soon as possible, and eat till your hearts are content!

Nutrition Facts
Calories: 250 calories, Proteins: 70 g, Carbs: 43 g, Fat: 10 g

Baked Potato Dish

Prep Time: 1 hour and 10 minutes/**Cook Time:** 45 minutes/**Servings:** 4/**Difficulty level:** Easy

Ingredients

- Kosher salt – according to your taste
- Russet potato – 1 Large
- Canola oil – according to your need

Instructions

1. The initial step is to warm the oven to 350 degrees Fahrenheit and place racks in the upper and lower thirds.
2. After doing that, perform a thorough cleaning of the potato (or potatoes) using a bristle brush and water flowing cold.
3. After the potato has been well dried, use a regular fork to make 8 to 12 large trench all over the surface of the spud. This will allow moisture to evaporate while the potato is being cooked.
4. Place inside a bowl and drizzle with oil to lightly coat.

5. Kosher salt should be used, and the potato should be placed directly on the rack in the center of the oven.
6. On the lowest rack, insert a baking sheet or a piece of aluminum foil to catch the drippings. People often like to use aluminum foil.
7. You should bake this for one hour or until the skin's surface is crisp, but the flesh beneath is still soft.
8. When you're ready to serve, use your fork to make a dotted line from one end to the other, and then crack open the potato by squeezing the two ends together. It will open in an instant. However, it would improve if you were careful because there would be steam.
9. If you are going to be cooking more than four potatoes at once, the cooking time will need to be increased by 15 minutes.

Nutrition Facts
Calories: 180 calories, Proteins: 70 g, Carbs: 59 g, Fat: 16 g

Black Bean Burrito

Cook Time: 30 minutes/**Servings:** 8/**Difficulty level:** Moderate

Ingredients

- Green chili pepper – 1 tablespoon minced fresh
- Lemon juice – 2 teaspoons
- Salt – 1 by 2 teaspoon
- Black beans - 4 cups cooked
- Broth - 2 teaspoons
- Salsa – fresh
- Onions - 3 cups diced
- Garlic cloves - 4 minced
- Cilantro leaf - 2/3 cup
- Coriander – 4 teaspoons
- Flour tortillas – 12
- Ground cumin - 4 teaspoons
- Sweet potatoes – 5 cups peeled cube

Instructions

1. The first step is to turn the oven temperature up to 350 degrees.
2. Put the potato in a medium-sized saucepan and cover them with water and salt.

3. The next thing to do is, bring the water to a boil.
4. Next, Cover the lid, bring to a boil, and then reduce heat to low and simmer for around ten minutes, or until the vegetables are soft.
5. Drain, then put it to the side.
6. While sweet potatoes boil, heat the oil in a medium saucepan or skillet and add the onions, garlic, and Chile.
7. On the other side, continue cooking until the onions are translucent.
8. Approximately seven minutes of cooking with the lid on and the heat set to medium-low, with occasional stirring, should be enough for the onions to become soft.
9. Cook for two to three minutes while tossing the mixture, often after adding the cumin and coriander.
10. Take the pan from the heat & put it to the side.
11. Combine the cooked sweet potatoes, black beans, cilantro, lemon juice, and salt in a food processor. Puree the mixture until smooth, and mash everything in a bowl by hand.
12. Move the sweet potato combination to a large bowl, and then stir in the onions and spices once they have finished cooking.
13. Prepare a big baking dish by lightly coating it in oil.
14. Set between two-thirds and three-quarters of a cup of the mixture in the middle of each wrap, roll up the tortilla, and place it in the casserole tray with the seam side down.
15. Bake for around thirty minutes, ensuring that the dish is thoroughly heated. Keep the foil tightly sealed over the top.
16. To serve, top each portion with salsa.

Nutrition Facts
Calories: 160 calories, Proteins: 83 g, Carbs: 69 g, Fat: 19 g

- Black pepper
- Lemon juice – 2 tablespoons
- Mayonnaise – 3 tablespoons
- Butter – 1 slice room temperature
- Green Onions – 3 tablespoons
- Seasoning salt – 1 by 4 teaspoon
- Tilapia fillets – 1 lb
- Parmesan cheese – 1 by 2 grated
- Basil – 1 by 4 teaspoon

Instructions
1. Preheat the oven to 375.
2. Dwelling the fillets in one layer in a baking dish or jellyroll pan measuring 13 by 9 inches and grease.
3. Do not stack fillets.
4. Coat the topping with the juice.
5. Cheese, butter, mayonnaise, onions, and seasonings should all be mixed in a bowl.
6. Stir thoroughly with a fork.
7. Fish should be baked in an oven that has been warmed for 10 to 20 minutes or until it begins to flake.
8. Banquet the cheese blend on top of the crackers, then bake for about 5 minutes or until the cheese mixture is golden brown.
9. The time necessary to bake the fish will be proportional to its thickness.
10. Keep a tight eye on the fish to ensure that this does not overcook.
11. Makes 4 servings.
12. Note that you may also cook this dish in the broiler.
13. Broil for 4 minutes or till almost done.
14. After adding the cheese, continue broiling for another two to three minutes or until the cheese has browned.

Nutrition Facts
Calories: 230 calories, Proteins: 70 g, Carbs: 34 g, Fat: 20 g

Super Tilapia Parmesan

Prep Time: 5 minutes/**Cook Time:** 35 minutes/**Servings:** 4/**Difficulty level:** Moderate

Ingredients
- Pepper sauce – 3 tablespoons

Pineapple and Ham Dinner

Preparation Time: 20 mins /**Cooking Time:** 15 mins /**Servings:** 4
Ingredients
- 2 ½ cups ham, cubed and cooked
- 2 tbsp butter
- 2 green chopped onions

- 1 ⅓ cups of pineapple juice
- 1 cup pineapple chunks
- 4 tsp cider vinegar
- 2 tsp prepared mustard
- 2 tbsp brown sugar
- 2 tbsp cornstarch

Directions
1. Melt the butter in a big skillet.
2. Saute the onions, pineapple chunks, and ham in the butter for approximately five minutes.
3. Mix the vinegar, pineapple juice, brown sugar, cornstarch, and mustard in a different medium-sized bowl.
4. Mix them well and spill over the ham mixture.
5. Stir and let it get thicken for about five minutes.
6. Serve.

Nutrition facts:
323 calories | protein 20g | carbohydrates 32.3g | fat 12.6g | sodium 1259mg

Savory Oatmeal with Mushrooms

Preparation Time: 15 mins / **Cooking Time:** 4 hours 10 minutes / **Servings:** 4
Ingredients:
- 1 cup steel-cut oats
- 8 ounces brown mushrooms, sliced
- 1/2 medium onion, chopped
- 1/2 teaspoon ground black pepper
- 1/2 teaspoon cayenne pepper
- 4 cups water
- 1/2 teaspoon sea salt
- 2 tablespoons grapeseed oil
- 4 cloves garlic, minced
- 3 sprigs of fresh thyme
- 1 cup baby spinach

Directions:
1. To 175 degrees F, preheat the sous vide water bath.
2. Place cooking pouches with steel-cut oats, water, salt, black pepper, and cayenne; seal firmly.
3. In the water bath, submerge the cooking pouches; boil for 4 hours; reserve.
4. Heat the oil in a pan preheated over a medium-high flame. Sauté, until softened, the mushrooms, onion, and garlic.
5. Now, add some new thyme and cook for another 5 minutes.
6. Spoon a blend of mushrooms over the cooked oatmeal.
7. Top with spinach for babies and serve wet.
8. Bon appétit!

Nutrition facts:
208 calories | protein 20.1g | carbohydrates 6.3g | fat 11.3g | sodium 243.5mg

Spice-Rubbed Ribs

Preparation Time: 10 mins / **Cooking Time:** 1 hour / **Servings:** 10
Ingredients
- 3 tbsp paprika
- 2 tbsp plus 1 tsp salt
- 2 tbsps plus
- 1 tsp garlic powder
- 2 tbsp cayenne pepper
- 4 tsp onion powder
- 4 tsp dried oregano
- 4 tsp dried thyme
- 4 tsp pepper
- 10 pounds of pork baby back ribs

Direction:
1. Combine the ingredients in a small dish; rub over the ribs.
2. Utilize a drip pan to prepare the grill for indirect cooking.
3. Grill ribs for 1 hour or until meat is cooked, flipping periodically.

Nutrition facts:
792 calories, 62g fat (23g saturated fat), 245mg cholesterol, 1864mg sodium, 5g carbohydrate (0 sugars, 2g fiber), 51g protein.

Chinese Pork Ribs

Preparation Time: 10 mins / **Cooking**

Time: 6 hours /**Servings:** 10
Ingredients:
- 1/4 cup of reduced-sodium soy sauce
- 1/3 cup of orange marmalade
- 3 tbsp ketchup
- 2 garlic cloves, minced
- 3 pounds bone-in country-style pork ribs

Direction:
1. Combine the soy sauce, marmalade, ketchup, and garlic in a small bowl.
2. Half of the mixture should be placed in a 5-quart slow cooker.
3. Add ribs to the top and sprinkle with leftover sauce.
4. Cook, covered, over low heat for 6-8 hours, or until the meat is cooked.
5. If desired, thicken cooking fluids.

Nutrition facts:
20g fat (7g saturated fat), 441 calories, 129mg cholesterol, 858mg sodium, 22g carbohydrate (19g sugars, 0 fiber), 40g protein.

Popcorn Shrimp

Preparation Time: 20 mins /**Cooking Time:** 15 minutes /**Servings:** 6
Ingredients:
- 1 pound small shrimp peeled and deveined
- 1 1/4 cups of all-purpose flour
- 2 tsp salt plus more for serving
- 1/2 tsp paprika smoked or regular
- 1/4 tsp pepper
- 1/4 tsp garlic powder
- 1 egg
- 1/4 cup of milk vegetable oil for frying
- 2 tsp chopped fresh parsley

Direction:
1. Combine the flour, salt, paprika, pepper, and garlic powder in a medium bowl.
2. To start, dry the shrimp and put them in a big bowl.
3. Toss in 1/4 cup of the flour mixture until all shrimp are coated.
4. Heat 3-4 inches of oil to 375 degrees F in a big deep pot.
5. Whisk together the egg and milk in a small bowl.
6. Each shrimp should be dipped into the milk mixture and dusted with the remaining seasoned flour.
7. 8-10 shrimp chunks in the oil Cook, occasionally stirring, for 2-3 minutes, or until golden brown.
8. To drain the shrimp, take them out of the oil and put them on a paper towel.
9. Rep with the remaining shrimp.
10. Serve immediately with chopped parsley.

Nutritions facts:
315kcal | Carbohydrates: 41g | Protein: 23g | Fat: 14g | Cholesterol: 271mg | Sodium: 677mg | Potassium: 408mg | Fiber: 1g

Lemon Rosemary Salmon

Preparation Time: 10 mins /**Cooking Time:** 20 minutes /**Servings:** 2
Ingredients
- 1 lemon, thinly sliced
- 4 sprigs of fresh rosemary
- 2 salmon fillets, bones, and skin removed
- coarse salt as needed
- 1 tbsp olive oil, or as needed

Direction:
1. Preheat the oven to 400°F oven
2. Arrange half of the lemon slices in a single layer in a baking dish.
3. Top with 2 rosemary sprigs and salmon fillets—Season salmon with salt and top with remaining rosemary sprigs and lemon wedges.
4. Drizzle with extra virgin olive oil.
5. Bake for twenty minutes, or until the fish is readily flaked with a fork.

Nutritions facts:
257 calories; protein 20.5g; carbohydrates 6.1g; fat 18g; cholesterol 56.4mg; sodium 1016.7mg.

Bowl Of Avocado And Tahini Paste

Preparation Time: 10 mins /**Cooking Time:** 0 minutes /**Servings:** 2

Ingredients
- 1 large avocado, destoned and diced
- 2 Tbsps (30 ml) of lime juice
- 2 Tbsps (30 ml) of olive oil, to cook with
- 2 cans of tuna (340 g), flaked
- 2 Tbsps of fresh cilantro, finely chopped
- 2 Tbsps (30 ml) of tahini sauce
- 3 Tbsps (45 ml) of gluten-free tamari sauce or coconut aminos
- 1 Tbsp (15 ml) of sesame oil

Direction:
1. To prepare the tahini tamari paste, thoroughly combine the paste's ingredients.
2. To prepare the tuna salad, whisk together the lime juice, cilantro, olive oil, and tuna.
3. To serve, spoon the avocado diced into a bowl and top with tuna and paste.

Nutrition facts:
Calories: 667, Fat: 48 g Carbohydrates: 15 g Fiber: 8 g Protein: 46 g, Sugar: 2 g

Cajun-spiced Tilapia

Preparation time: 5 mins/**Cooking time:** 5 mins /**Servings:** 2

Ingredients:
- 8 oz tilapia fillets
- ½ tsp Chinese five-spice powder
- 2 tbsp reduced-sodium soy sauce
- 1 tbsp granulated stevia
- 2 tsps olive oil
- 1 cup sugar snap peas
- 2 scallions, thinly sliced

Directions:
1. Sprinkle both sides of the fillets with the Chinese five-spice powder.
2. In a small bowl, stir together the soy sauce and stevia.
3. Set aside.
4. Heat the olive oil in a large nonstick skillet set over medium-high heat.
5. Add the tilapia.
6. Cook for about 2 mins, or until the outer edges are opaque.
7. Reduce the heat to medium.
8. Turn the fish over.
9. Stir the soy mixture and pour into the skillet.
10. Add the sugar snap peas.
11. Bring the sauce to a boil.
12. Cook for about 2 mins, or until the fish is cooked through, the sauce thickens, and the peas are bright green.
13. Add scallions.
14. Remove from the heat.
15. Serve the fish and the sugar snap peas drizzled with the pan sauce.

Nutrition Facts:
calories 202, fat 7g, Protein 26g, carbs 7g, sugars 3g, fiber 0g, sodium 619mg

Tuna Melts

Preparation time: 5 mins/**Cooking time:** 5 mins /**Servings:** 3

Ingredients:
- 3 English muffins, 100% whole-wheat
- 2 (5-ounce) cans tuna, drained
- 2 tbsp plain Greek yogurt
- ½ tsp freshly ground black pepper
- ¾ cup shredded cheddar cheese

Directions:
1. If your broiler is at the top of your oven, place the oven rack in the center.
2. Turn the broiler on high.
3. Split the English muffins, if necessary, and toast them in the toaster.
4. Meanwhile, in a medium bowl, mix the tuna, yogurt, and pepper.
5. Place the muffin halves on a baking sheet, and spoon one-sixth of the tuna mixture and 2 tbsp of cheddar cheese on top of each half.

6. Broil for 2 mins or until the cheese melts.

Nutrition Facts:
calories 392, fat 13g, Protein 40g, carbs 28g, sugars 6g, fiber 5g, sodium 474mg

Grilled Cod

Preparation time: 5 mins/**Cooking Time:** 10 mins/**Servings:** 4
Ingredients:
- 2 (8 ounces) fillets of cod, cut in half
- 1 tbsp oregano
- ½ tsp lemon pepper
- ¼ tsp ground black pepper
- 2 tbsps olive oil
- 1 lemon, juiced
- 2 tbsps chopped green onion (white part only)

Directions:
1. Season both sides of cod with oregano, lemon pepper, and black pepper.
2. Set fish aside on a plate.
3. Green onion and butter are heated in a small saucepan over medium heat. Lemon juice and butter are then added, and the onion is cooked for about 3 minutes.
4. Place cod on oiled grill grates and cook for about 3 minutes on each side, or until fish flakes easily. During cooking, baste cod regularly with the olive oil mixture.
5. Before serving, let the fish rest for about 5 minutes off the heat.

Nutrition facts:
calories 92, fat 7.4g, sodium 19mg, carbs 2.5g, fiber 1g, Protein 5.4g, potassium 50mg, phosphorus 36 mg

Cod and Green Bean Curry

Preparation time: 10 mins/**Cooking Time:** 60 mins/**Servings:** 4
Ingredients:
- 1/2-pound green beans, trimmed and cut into bite-sized pieces
- 1 white onion, sliced
- 2 cloves garlic, minced
- 1 tbsp olive oil, or more as needed

Curry Mixture:
- 2 tbsp water, or more as needed
- 2 tsp curry powder
- 2 tsp ground ginger
- 1 1/2 (6 ounces) cod fillets

Directions:
1. Preheat the oven to 400 °F.
2. Combine green beans, onion, and garlic in a large glass baking dish.
3. Toss with olive oil to coat; season with pepper.
4. Bake in the oven, occasionally stirring, until the edges of the onion are slightly charred and the green beans start to look dry, about 40 mins.
5. In the meantime, mix water, curry powder, and ginger.
6. Remove the dish and stir the vegetables; stir in the curry mixture.
7. Increase oven temperature to 450°F.
8. Put the vegetables on top of the cod and place it in the bottom of the dish.
9. Continually bake the fish for 25 to 30 minutes, depending on thickness, until it is opaque.

Nutrition Facts:
calories 64, fat 3.8g, sodium 5mg, carbs 7.7g, fiber 2.9g, Protein 1.6g, potassium 180mg, phosphorus 101 mg

Calamari Salad

Preparation time: 5 mins/**Cooking Time:** 0 mins/**Servings:** 2
Ingredients:
- 1 peeled and sliced cucumber
- lettuce leaves
- 3 ½ oz. washed, cleaned, and sliced calamari fillets
- fresh parsley, chopped
- 1 peeled, boiled, and sliced potato
- 1 tbsp sour cream
- 1 peeled, cored, and sliced apple

Directions:

1. Place the calamari into boiling salted water and cook for 5 min.
2. Arrange lettuce leaves on the bottom of a salad bowl.
3. Mix the apple and vegetable strips with the calamari.
4. Dress in sour cream, place on the lettuce leaves, and garnish with the parsley.

Nutrition facts:
calories 468, fat 8g, sodium 49mg, carbs 5.4g, fiber 1.3g, Protein 17g, potassium 142mg, phosphorus 151 mg

Acorn Squash with Stuffing

Prep time: 5 mins /**Cook time:** 10 mins /**Serving:** 2
Ingredients:
- Squash acorns
- 2 peeled and chopped apples
- 1/2 cup brown stevia
- A quarter teaspoon of cinnamon
- Nutmeg (1/4 teaspoon)
- Lemon juice, 2 tablespoons
- 1/4 cup unsalted butter

Directions:
1. Cut the squash in half lengthwise, then scoop out the seeds.
2. Evenly distribute the diced apple among the squash halves.
3. Sprinkle a quarter of the brown stevia, cinnamon, nutmeg, and a few drops of lemon juice over each half.
4. 1 tablespoon (14 g) butter, a dot on each.
5. Wrap each squash half in foil tightly.
6. Fill the slow cooker with 1/4 cup (60 milliliters) of water.
7. Stack the squash in the cooker, and cut the side up.
8. Cook on low for 5 hours, covered.
9. Unwrap the squash and arrange it on a serving plate.

Nutritional facts:
168 calories, 10 g fat, 13 g carbs, 11 g protein

Mussels Steamed in Coconut Broth

Prep time: 10 mins /**Cook time:** 10 mins /**Serving:** 2
Ingredients:
- 2 tablespoons unsalted butter
- 1 cup chopped shallots
- garlic cloves, minced
- 2 teaspoons seasoning (Italian)
- 1 tbsp. stevia extract
- 1 cup tomatoes, cherry
- mussels, 2 lbs., cleaned and rinsed
- 1 quart of coconut milk
- 1 tbsp. tapioca flour

Directions:
1. In the Instant Pot, melt the butter in sauté mode.
2. Cook until the shallots are tender (approximately 2 minutes)
3. Stir in the garlic and simmer until fragrant (about 1 minute.)
4. Add the cherry tomatoes and cook, constantly stirring, until the sauce boils.
5. Return to a boil with the remaining ingredients (excluding the finishing ingredients).
6. Add the mussels and stir until everything is well mixed.
7. Close and lock the lid.
8. Change the vent's setting to Sealing.
9. Cook for 6 minutes on high pressure.
10. In a small dish, mix the coconut milk and tapioca starch.
11. Pour the milk mixture into the Instant Pot and stir until the soup thickens.

Nutritional facts:
163 calories, 10 g fat, 13 g carbs, 11 g protein

Caramelized Onions

Prep time: 10 mins /**Cook time:** 10 mins /**Serving:** 2
Ingredients:
- 6 big sweet onions
- 1/4 cup (55 g) butter
- 1/4 cup (285 ml) chicken broth

Directions:
1. Onions should be peeled.
2. Remove the root ends and stems.
3. Put everything in the slow cooker.
4. Butter and broth should be poured over the onions.
5. Cook for 12 hours on low.

Nutritional facts:
162 calories, 10 g fat, 13 g carbs, 11 g protein
Glycemic Index: Low 6.4

Italian Style Stuffed Tomatoes

Prep time: 10 mins /**Cook time:** 10 mins /**Serving:** 2
Ingredients:
- 4 cups cooked navy beans (drained and rinsed)
- 1/2 moderate yellow onion, peeled and sliced tiny
- artichoke hearts (oil-free), drained and coarsely chopped
- 6 big tomatoes (beefsteak, for example)

Directions:
1. In a small bowl, mix the beans, artichoke hearts, onion, and pesto; put aside.
2. Cut a 12-inch slice from the top of each tomato and scoop off the meat, leaving a 12-inch shell.

Nutritional facts:
161 calories, 10 g fat, 13 g carbs, 11 g protein.

Greek Green Beans & Tomatoes

Prep time: 10 mins /**Cook time:** 10 mins /**Serving:** 2
Ingredients:
- Fresh green beans,
- 1 pound 1 mug (235 ml) chopped tomatoes with no salt added
- 1 mug (160 g) onion, chopped
- 1/2 teaspoon oregano, dry
- 1 tsp. lemon extract

- 1 tablespoon (15 ml) extra virgin olive oil
- To taste black pepper

Directions:
1. In a slow cooker, mix all of the ingredients.
2. Stir. Cook on low for 6 hours, covered.

Nutritional facts:
188 calories, 10 g fat, 13 g carbs, 11 g protein
Glycemic Index: Low 6.6

Orange Flavored Carrots

Prep time: 10 mins /**Cook time:** 15 mins /**Serving:** 2
Ingredients:
- quarts liquid
- 1 pound peeled and sliced carrots
- 1 1/2 tablespoons orange zest, grated
- tbsp. spread like margarine
- 2 tbsp. dark brown stevia, packed
- 1 teaspoon mustard (Dijon)
- Salt (1/4 teaspoon)

Directions:
1. Fill a big saucepan halfway with water.
2. In a saucepan, place the foldable steamer basket.
3. Carrots should be arranged in a basket.
4. Bring to a boil, coated, over high heat.
5. Cook for 8 minutes or until carrots is crisp and tender.
6. Remove the carrots from the steamer basket and mix them with the other ingredients in a moderate mixing dish.

Nutritional facts:
296 calories, 13 g fat, 16 g carbs, 24 g protein
Glycemic Index: Low 6.7

Basic Lima Beans

Prep time: 10 mins /**Cook time:** 10 mins /**Serving:** 2
Ingredients:
- Dried lima beans,
- 1 pound (455 g)
- 12 cup chopped onion (240 g)
- 12 cup celery, chopped (50 g)

- big peeled and chopped potatoes
- 1 cup sliced carrots (130 g)

Directions:
1. Wash the beans and put them in the slow cooker with the rest of the ingredients.

Nutritional facts:
195 calories, 10 g fat, 13 g carbs, 11 g protein

Egg and Salsa

Prep. Time: 5 mins /**Cooking Time:** 5 mins /**Serving:** 4
Ingredients:
- 1 egg
- 2 tbsp oil
- 3 tbsp salsa
- ½ avocado sliced
- 10 crushed tortilla chips
- 2 cups mesclun
- 1 tbsp cilantro
- 200 g cooked kidney beans

Direction:
2. Mix the salsa with cilantro and 1 tbsp olive oil.
3. Put the mesclun in a large salad bowl and pour half the salsa mix into the mesclun.
4. Next, place the kidney beans and avocado slices on top.
5. Next, put a layer of chips.
6. Then fry a sunny egg side up, and put it on top of the salad bed.
7. Enjoy your dinner.

Nutritional facts:
Calories: 148 kcal Carbohydrates: 6.7 g Proteins: 3.3 g Fats: 13 g Sodium: 27 mg

Chapter 13: Dessert Recipe

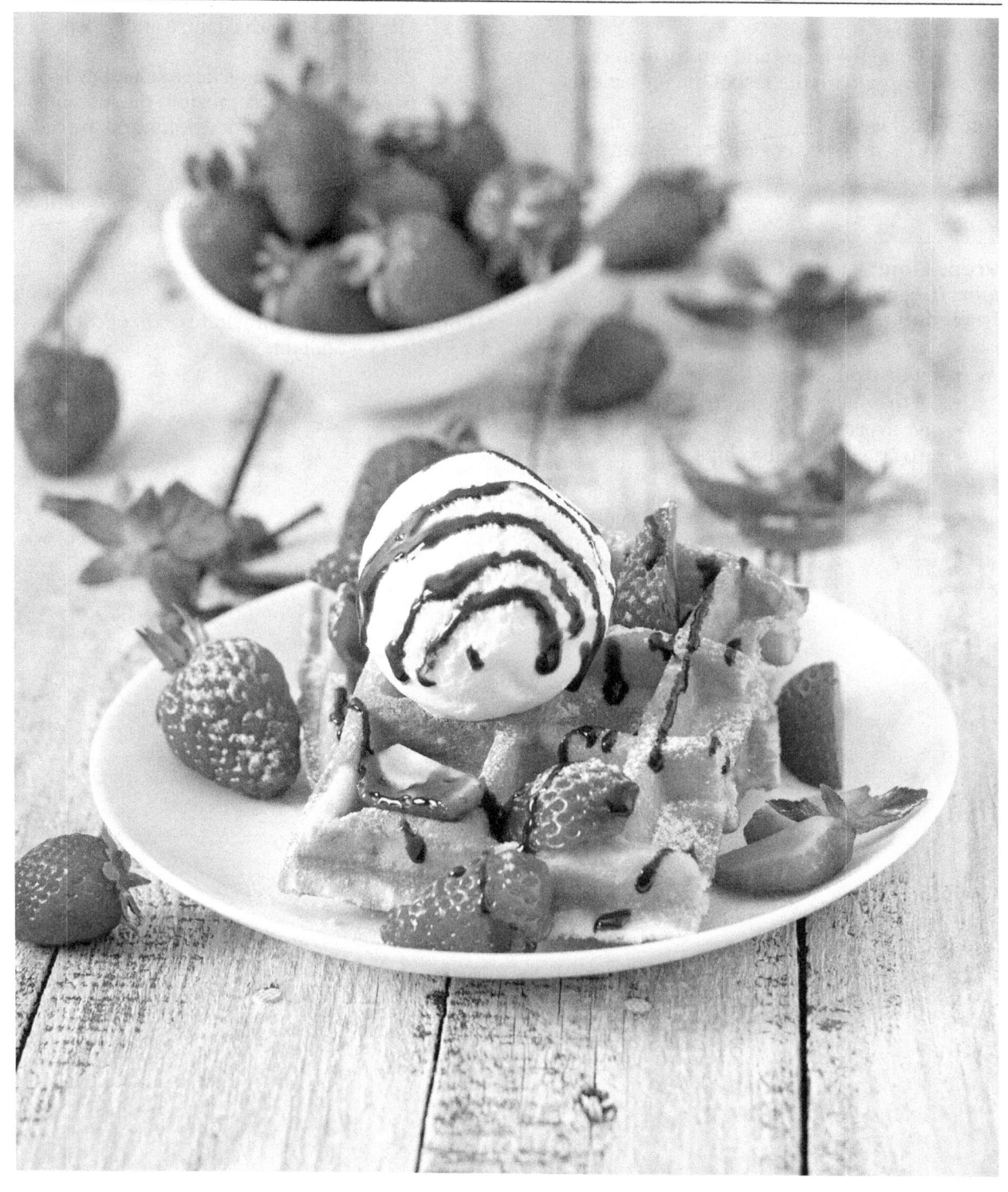

Banana Ice-Cream

Prep Time: 5 mins /**Cooking Time:** N/A' /**Serving Size:** 3
Ingredients:
- 3 frozen bananas

Direction:
1. Peel and slice the bananas and store them in a zip lock bag in a freezer for 3 hours.
2. Take out from the freezer, add to a food processor, and start pulsing at the highest speed.
3. After 3 to 4 mins, you will see that the pieces will start to form chunks.
4. Next, open the processor and scrape the bananas from the corners.
5. Again, start pulsing, and the banana will form oatmeal consistency.
6. Again, scrape the mango from the corners.
7. Keep pulsing, and you will see a creamy texture starts forming.
8. Blend for 2 more minutes and scoop the ice cream.
9. Enjoy your 1 ingredient ice cream.

Nutritional facts:
Calories: 106 kcal Carbohydrates: 25 g Protein: 1.3 g Fats: 0.4 g Sodium: 1 mg

Cottage Cheese and Fruit Snacks

Prep Time: 5 mins /**Cooking Time:** N/A /**Serving:** 4
Ingredients:
- ½ cup cut apples
- ½ cup cut kiwi
- 2 cut strawberries
- 5 blueberries
- 50 g crumbled cottage cheese

Direction:
1. In a mixing bowl, mix all ingredients.
2. Enjoy your sweet snack.

Nutritional facts:
Calories: 179 kcal Carbohydrates: 32 g Protein: 6 g Fats: 5 g Sodium: 80 mg

Protein Bars

Prep Time: 5 mins /**Cooking Time:** N/A /**Serving:** 5
Ingredients:
- ½ cup almonds
- 1 cup pitted dates
- ¼ tsp salt substitute
- 1 tsp vanilla extract
- ½ cup cashew nuts
- 25 g flax seeds
- 25 g chia seeds

Direction:
1. Add all ingredients to a food processor and mix till a smooth mixture is formed.
2. Now take out the mixture and divide it into 12 parts.
3. Make balls and keep them in the refrigerator.
4. Use one at a time.
5. These can be kept for up to 2 weeks.

Nutritional facts:
Calories: 131 kcal Carbohydrates: 18 g Protein: 3.4 g Fats: 7.3 g Sodium: 3 mg

Raspberry Jelly

Prep Time: 10 mins /**Cooking Time:** 10 mins /**Serving:** 4
Ingredients:
- 1 cup raspberries
- 4 tbsp honey
- 1 tsp gelatin
- 2 cups water

Direction:
1. In a blender, blend water and raspberries.
2. Now heat this mixture in a saucepan.

3. Add gelatin and cook for two more minutes.
4. Add honey and mix well. Put into molds and cool till the jelly sets.

Nutritional facts:
Calories: 86 kcal Carbohydrates: 21 g Protein: 1.9 g Fats: 0.2 g Sodium: 8 mg

Cheesecake

Prep time: 15 mins /**Cooking time:** 1 hour 25 min /**Serving:** 4
Ingredients:
- 2 cups graham cracker crumbs
- 3 eggs
- 600g cream cheese
- 150g sour cream
- 1/3 cup cream
- 1 ½ tbsp lemon rind
- 1/3 cup unsalted butter
- 1 cup sugar
- 1 tsp vanilla essence

Direction:
1. Preheat the oven to 225°F.
2. Mix melted butter, graham cracker crumbs, sugar, and press into the removable pan in a bowl.
3. Bake for 10 minutes.
4. After removing the pan and letting it cool fully, turn off the oven.
5. Using an electric mixer, combine the sugar and cream cheese.
6. Mix in the sour cream, lemon rind, and vanilla after adding them.
7. Blend in the cream and eggs after adding them.
8. Fill the springform pan with liquid.
9. Cover the entire springform pan with plastic wrap and wrap it in the container twice.
10. The cling wrap should cover the pan thoroughly.
11. Place the pan into the oven.
12. Set the oven to Convection Mode at 225°F. Bake for 1 hour and 15 minutes

Nutritional facts:
Calories: 516 kcal Carbohydrates: 64 g Protein: 6.6 g Fats: 28 g Sodium: 255 mg

Beans Brownies

Preparation time: 15 min /**Cooking time:** 15 min /**Servings:** 6
Ingredients:
- 1 cup black beans, cooked
- 1 tablespoon cocoa powder
- 5 oz quick oats
- 3 tablespoons of liquid honey
- 1 teaspoon baking powder
- 1 tablespoon lemon juice
- 1 teaspoon vanilla extract
- 1 teaspoon olive oil

Directions:
1. Mash black beans until smooth and stir with cocoa powder, honey, quick oats, baking powder, lemon juice, and vanilla extract.
2. Add olive oil and stir with the spoon.
3. Then, cover the baking pan with baking paper.
4. Transfer the brownie mixture to the baking tray and flatten it well.
5. Cut the brownie into the bars.
6. Bake the dessert in the preheated to 360F oven for 15 minutes.
7. Cool the cooked brownies well.

Nutrition facts:
Calories 82; Fat 3 g; Saturated Fat 1 g; Carbs 8 g; Sugars 0 g; Fiber 3 g; Protein 4 g; Cholesterol 40 mg; Sodium 45 mg; Potassium 130 mg

Avocado Mousse

Preparation time: 10 min /**Cooking time:** 0 min /**Servings:** 2
Ingredients:
- 1 avocado, peeled, pitted
- ½ cup low-fat milk
- 1 teaspoon vanilla extract
- 1 tablespoon cocoa powder
- 2 teaspoons liquid honey

Directions:

- Chop avocado and put it in the food processor.
- Add milk, vanilla extract, and cocoa powder.
- Blend the mixture until smooth.
- Pour the cooked mousse into the jar and top with honey.

Nutrition facts: Calories 174; Fat 9 g; Saturated Fat 2 g; Carbs 11 g; Sugars 0 g; Fiber 7 g; Protein 4 g; Cholesterol 0 mg; Sodium 30 mg; Potassium 330 mg

Fruit Kebabs

Preparation time: 10 min /**Cooking time:** 0 min /**Servings:** 3
Ingredients:
- 1 cup strawberries
- 1 cup melon, cubed
- 1 cup grapes
- 2 kiwis, cubed
- 1 cup watermelon, cubed

Directions:
1. String the fruits in the wooden skewers one by one.
2. Put the cooked fruit kebabs in the fridge for 30 minutes.

Nutrition facts:
Calories 54; Fat 0 g; Saturated Fat 0 g; Carbs 10 g; Sugars 3 g; Fiber 1.4 g; Protein 1.8 g; Cholesterol 0 mg; Sodium 10 mg; Potassium 130 mg

Vanilla Soufflé

Preparation time: 10 min /**Cooking time:** 30 min /**Servings:** 2
Ingredients:
- 2 egg yolks, whisked
- 2 tablespoons whole-grain wheat flour
- 1 teaspoon vanilla extract
- 1 tablespoon potato starch
- 2 tablespoons agave nectar
- 1 cup of low-fat milk

1. **Directions:**
2. Mix up milk and egg yolks.
3. Add vanilla extract, flour, and potato starch.
4. Mix the liquid until smooth and bring it to a boil.
5. Add agave syrup and stir well.
6. Then spread the mixture into the soufflé ramekins and transfer them to the preheated 350F oven.
7. Bake soufflé for 17 minutes.

Nutrition facts:
Calories 105; Fat 1 g; Saturated Fat 0 g; Carbs 15 g; Sugars 7 g; Fiber 0 g; Protein 4 g; Cholesterol 4 mg; Sodium 65 mg; Potassium 10 mg

Strawberries in Dark Chocolate

Preparation time: 15 min /**Cooking time:** 1 min /**Servings:** 2
Ingredients:
- 1 cup strawberries
- 1 tablespoon olive oil
- 1 oz dark chocolate, chopped

Directions:
1. Put the chocolate in the microwave oven for 30 seconds and melt it.
2. Then mix up olive oil and chocolate.
3. Whisk well.
4. Freeze the strawberries for 15 minutes.
5. Then sprinkle them with a chocolate mixture.

Nutrition facts:
Calories 141; Fat 4.4 g; Saturated Fat 0 g; Carbs 20 g; Sugars 8 g; Fiber 0 g; Protein 0 g; Cholesterol 10 mg; Sodium 0 mg; Potassium 180 mg

White bean dip

Preparation Time: 10 minutes /**Cooking Time:** 0 minutes /**Servings:** 4
Ingredients:
- Zest of ¼ lemon
- 2 tablespoons olive oil
- 15 ounces canned beans, drained and rinsed
- 5-6 canned artichoke hearts, drained and quartered
- 3 garlic cloves, minced
- 1 tablespoon basil, chopped
- Juice of ¼ lemon
- Salt & black pepper to taste

Directions:
1. Pulse together the beans, artichokes, and the remaining ingredients in a food processor, excluding the oil.
2. Gradually add the oil, pulse the mixture once more, divide into cups, and serve as a party dip.

Nutrition facts:
Calories 27 kcal, Fat 11.7g, Carbs 18.5g, Sugar 2g, Protein 16.5g 183

Hummus with ground lamb

Preparation Time: 10 minutes /**Cooking Time:** 15 minutes /**Servings:** 8
Ingredients:
- 10 ounces hummus
- 12 ounces lamb meat, ground
- ½ cup pomegranate seeds
- ¼ cup parsley, chopped
- 1 tablespoon olive oil
- Pita chips for serving

Directions:
1. In a pan heated over medium heat, brown the meat for 15 minutes while stirring frequently.
2. Spread hummus on a platter, top with ground lamb, sprinkle with pomegranate seeds and parsley, and serve with pita chips as an appetizer.

Nutrition facts:
Calories 133 kcal, Fat 9.7g, Carbs 6.4g, Sugar 10g, Protein 5.4g

Eggplant dip

Preparation Time: 10 minutes /**Cooking Time:** 40 minutes /**Servings:** 4
Ingredients:
- 1 eggplant, poked with a fork
- 2 tablespoons tahini paste
- 1 tablespoon parsley, chopped
- 1 tablespoon lemon juice
- 2 tablespoon olive oil
- 3 garlic cloves, crushed
- Salt and black pepper to taste

Directions:
1. The eggplant should be placed in a roasting pan, baked for 40 minutes at 400 °F, let to cool, then peeled and added to your food processor.
2. The other ingredients, minus the parsley, should be blended and pulsed well before being divided into small bowls and served as an appetizer with some parsley on top.

Nutrition facts:
Calories 121 kcal, Fat 4.3g, Carbs 1.4g, Sugar 2g, Protein 4.3g

Veggie fritters

Preparation Time: 10 minutes /**Cooking Time:** 10 minutes /**Servings:** 8
Ingredients:
- 3 garlic cloves, minced
- 2 yellow onions, chopped
- 2 scallions, chopped
- 2 carrots, grated
- 2 teaspoons cumin, ground
- ½ teaspoon turmeric powder
- Salt and black pepper to the taste
- ¼ teaspoon coriander, ground
- 1 tablespoons parsley, chopped
- ¼ teaspoon lemon juice
- ½ cup almond flour
- 2 beets, peeled and grated

- 2 eggs, whisked
- ¼ cup tapioca flour
- 2 tablespoons olive oil

Directions:
1. In a bowl, combine the garlic with the onions, scallions, and the remaining ingredients, excluding the oil, and stir until well combined.
2. Preheat the pan over medium-high heat, place the fritters, cook for 5 minutes on each side, arrange on a platter and serve.

Nutrition facts:
Calories 209 kcal, Fat 11.2g, Carbs 4.4g, Sugar 2.7g, Protein 4.8g

Bulgur lamb meatballs

Preparation Time: 10 minutes /**Cooking Time:** 15 minutes /**Servings:** 6
Ingredients:
- 1 and ½ cups Greek yogurt
- ½ teaspoon cumin, ground
- 1 cup cucumber, shredded
- ½ teaspoon garlic, minced
- A pinch of salt and black pepper
- 1 cup bulgur
- 2 cups water
- 1-pound lamb, ground
- ¼ cup parsley, chopped
- ¼ cup shallots, chopped
- ½ teaspoon allspice, ground
- ½ teaspoon cinnamon powder
- 1 tablespoon olive oil

Directions:
1. Combine the bulgur and water in a bowl, cover, set aside for 10 minutes, then drain and transfer to another bowl.
2. Add the meat, yogurt, and the remaining ingredients, excluding the oil, and mix thoroughly.
3. Form medium-sized meatballs from this mixture.
4. Preheat the pan over medium-high heat, place the meatballs, cook them for 7 minutes on each side, arrange them on a platter and serve as an appetizer.

Nutrition facts:
Calories 300 kcal, Fat 9.6g, Carbs 22.6g, Sugar 4g, Protein 6.6g

Baked apricot dessert

Preparation Time: 10 minutes /**Cooking Time:** 15 minutes /**Servings:** 1
Ingredients:
- Melted butter for greasing
- 1 825g can apricot halves, drained
- 50g (1/3 cup) self-raising flour
- 110g (1/2 cup) caster sugar
- 1 tsp vanilla essence
- 2 eggs, lightly whisked
- 1 200g carton natural yogurt
- 1 300g carton sour cream
- Pinch ground nutmeg

Directions:
1. Heat the oven to 190°C. To gently oil a 1.75-1itre (7-cup) ovenproof dish, brush it with melted butter.
2. Arrange the apricots, rounded side up, on the bottom of the prepared plate.
3. In a large mixing bowl, sift the flour.
4. Combine the caster sugar, vanilla extract, eggs, yogurt, and sour cream in a mixing bowl. Whisk until everything is thoroughly blended.
5. Pour the sour cream and apricot mixture over the apricots.
6. Garnish with nutmeg.
7. Bake for 20-25 minutes, or until just set, in a preheated oven.
8. Spoon into dishes and serve right away.

Nutrition facts:
Calories 305 kcal, Fat 9.7g, Carbs 22.2g, Sugar 6g, Protein 6.9g

Blackberry chocolate dessert cake

Preparation Time: 10 minutes /**Cooking Time:** 15 minutes /**Servings:** 1
Ingredients:
- 250g butter, chopped
- 250g of good-quality dark chocolate, chopped

- 1/3 cup milk
- 1 cup caster sugar
- 4 eggs, at room temperature, separated
- 1/3 cup plain flour
- 150g frozen blackberries
- Solid chocolate Easter eggs to serve
- Extra blackberries to serve
- Cocoa powder, to serve

Directions:
1. Heat the oven to 200°C. Line a 23cm springform pan with baking paper and grease it.
2. In a small saucepan over medium heat, properly melt the butter.
3. Place aside.
4. In a large heatproof dish, combine the chocolate and milk.
5. Place the bowl over a pot of simmering water (do not allow the bottom of the bowl to touch the water).
6. Stirring constantly with a metal spoon, heat until melted and smooth.
7. Beat in the sugar using an electric hand mixer.
8. Remove the dish from the heat.
9. Allow for a 10-minute cooling period.
10. One at a time, add egg yolks to the chocolate mixture, beating well after each addition.
11. Put the melted butter in.
12. Mix everything together by stirring.
13. Flour should be sifted over the chocolate mixture.
14. Fold in gently.
15. In a separate dish, whisk the egg whites until soft peaks form.
16. Fold gently into the chocolate mixture.
17. Garnish with blackberries.
18. Fold in gently until incorporated.
19. Pour the ingredients into the prepared pan.
20. Bake for 15 minutes, or until the cake has risen.
21. Reduce the oven temperature to 160°C.
22. Bake for 45 minutes more, or until a skewer inserted into the center comes clean.
23. Allow it cool entirely in the pan (don't worry if the cake sinks in the center).
24. Place the cake properly on a dish to serve.
25. Chocolate eggs and blackberries can be used to decorate.
26. Dust with chocolate powder.
27. If desired, top slices with mascarpone or heavy cream.

Nutrition facts:
Calories 315 kcal, Fat 9.9g, Carbs 23.2g, Sugar 7g, Protein 6.9g

Layered mascarpone & strawberry dessert

Preparation Time: 10 minutes / **Cooking Time:** 15 minutes / **Servings:** 1

Ingredients:
- 500g (2 punnets) strawberries, hulled
- 60ml (1/4 cup) blackcurrant liqueur (creme de cassis)
- 115g (1/2 cup) caster sugar
- 1 250g container mascarpone
- 125ml (1/2 cup) thickened cream

Directions:
1. Cut 250g (1 punnet) strawberries in halves and combine with 2 tablespoons liqueur in a dish. To mix, toss everything together.
2. Set aside to macerate, covered.
3. Place the remaining strawberries in a small saucepan with the remaining liquor and sugar. Over medium heat, stir until the sugar melts.
4. Cook for 6-7 minutes, or until the strawberries soften, stirring regularly.
5. Blend the strawberry mixture in a blender or food processor bowl until smooth.
6. Transfer to a basin, cover, and refrigerate for 1 hour, or until the mixture is well cooled.
7. In a medium mixing basin, whisk together the mascarpone and cream with a balloon whisk until the mascarpone thickens (it will become thinner at first before thickening again - take care not to over whisk).
8. Next, whisk in the strawberry mixture until it thickens slightly.

9. One-third of the mascarpone mixture should be divided among four 250ml (1-cup) serving glasses.
10. Add a third of the macerated strawberries on top.
11. The remaining mascarpone mixture and macerated strawberries are repeated to produce two additional layers.
12. Serve right away. **Nutrition facts:**

Calories 321 kcal, Fat 9.3g, Carbs 24.2g, Sugar 7g, Protein 6.5g

Spiced apple dessert

Preparation Time: 10 minutes /**Cooking Time:** 15 minutes /**Servings:** 1
Ingredients:
- 1 cup self-raising flour
- 1/2 tbsp caster sugar
- 30g butter, chilled, chopped
- Pinch of salt
- 1/3 cup buttermilk
- 1 small granny smith apple
- Buttermilk, extra, for brushing
- 1/3 cup brown sugar
- 1/2 tsp mixed spice

Directions:
1. Set the oven to 200 degrees fan-forced.
2. the oven to 350 °F. Use parchment paper to cover a baking sheet.
3. The upper portion of the oven should contain the oven rack.
4. In a mixing bowl, sift the flour, sugar, and salt.
5. Melted butter should be added.
6. With your hands, incorporate the butter into the flour mixture until it resembles fine breadcrumbs.
7. In the center of the mixture, make a well.
8. Add the buttermilk.
9. Using a flat-bladed knife, stir until a sticky dough forms.
10. Place the dough on a lightly floured board and roll it out.
11. Knead the dough carefully until it is smooth.
12. Roll out the dough until it is 2cm thick, using a lightly floured rolling pin. Scones should be cut out with a 7cm circular cutter.
13. Combine any remaining dough. Make 4 scones in total.
14. Place one apple in the bottom of four 1/2 cup ramekins.
15. Season with sugar and spice.
16. Place the scones in ramekins and top with the sugar mixture.
17. Brush the tops with more buttermilk.
18. Arrange ramekins on a tray.
19. Bake for 10 minutes until the top is light brown and the sugar bubbles around the edges.
20. Set aside for 4 minutes before transferring to plates.
21. Serve.

Nutrition facts:
Calories 333 kcal, Fat 8.7g, Carbs 23.2g, Sugar 6g, Protein 6.9g

Apple crumble dessert cake

Preparation Time: 10 minutes /**Cooking Time:** 15 minutes /**Servings:** 1
Ingredients:
- 220g butter, chopped, melted
- 4 eggs, at room temperature
- 2 3/4 cups self-raising flour
- 1 1/2 cups caster sugar
- 1 cup sour cream
- 1/3 cup Foster Clark's custard powder
- 1 tsp vanilla essence
- 800g can eat apple pie fruit
- Double thick cream to serve
- 3/4 cup plain flour
- 1/3 cup white sugar
- 1 tsp baking powder
- 1 tsp ground cinnamon
- 75g butter, chilled, chopped

Directions:
1. Melted butter, eggs, flour, caster sugar, sour cream, custard powder, and vanilla extract should be mixed for 3 minutes or until pale and frothy.
2. Half of the mixture should be poured into the prepared dish or pan.
3. Spread the apple over the mixture.

4. Finish with the remaining mixture.
5. Combine the flour, white sugar, baking powder, and cinnamon in a mixing dish.
6. Rub the butter into the flour mixture with your hands until it resembles coarse breadcrumbs.
7. Sprinkle topping on top of the cake mixture.
8. 1 hour to 1 hour 15 minutes, or until a skewer inserted into the center comes out clean.
9. Serve with cream while still warm.

Nutrition facts:
Calories 340 kcal, Fat 8.7g, Carbs 23.2g, Sugar 8g, Protein 6.5g

Chapter 14 - 21 Days Meal Plan

MEAL PLAN

Sun			
Mon			
Tue			
Wed			
Thu			
Fri			
Sat			

Days	Breakfast	Lunch	Dinner
1	Pumpkin-Peanut Butter Single-Serve Muffins	Pepper and Pesto Chicken Panini	Sweetened Potato Curry with Chickpeas
2	Breakfast Sausage Casserole	Mashed Cauliflower	Pineapple and Ham Dinner
3	Crustless Broccoli Cheese Quiche	Bum's Lunch	Savory Oatmeal with Mushrooms
4	Fruits Breakfast Salad	High-Temp Pork Roast	Spice-Rubbed Ribs
5	Pesto Egg Casserole	Chickpea Salad with Tomato and Red Onion	Chinese Pork Ribs
6	Kiwi Shake	Chicken & Bacon Caesar Salad	Popcorn Shrimp
7	Greek Toast	Barbecued Poussins with Chili Corn Salsa	Lemon Rosemary Salmon
8	Mushrooms Bites	Kale Lasagna with Meat Sauce	Bowl Of Avocado And Tahini Paste
9	Whole-Grain Pancakes	Blue Cheese, Spinach Meat Loaf Muffins	Cajun-spiced Tilapia
10	Omelet with Asparagus	Syrian Rice with Meat	Tuna Melts
11	Breakfast Granola	Deer Meat	Grilled Cod
12	Breakfast Egg Toasts	Sicilian Meat Roll	Cod and Green Bean Curry
13	Ricotta Toast with Pistachios and Honey	Chicken-Apricot Casserole	Calamari Salad
14	Granny Smith Apples	Pasta with grilled chicken, white beans, and mushrooms	Acorn Squash with Stuffing
15	Spiced Congee with Dates	Lemon Rosemary Chicken	Mussels Steamed in Coconut Broth
16	Ham and Cheddar Omelets	Chicken Zucchini Pie	Caramelized Onions
17	Basic Oatmeal	Chicken Etouffee	Italian Style Stuffed Tomatoes
18	Chorizo, Tomato & Grill Chili Frittata	Tasty Fish Fillets	Greek Green Beans & Tomatoes
19	Muesli with Coconut, Oats & Bananas	Grilled Dory Fish	Orange Flavored Carrots
20	Steel-Cut Oats	Tuna and Broccoli Pasta	Basic Lima Beans
21	Keto Turmeric Milkshake	Chicken with Herbs	Egg and Salsa

Conclusion

The theory behind fasting is that if we reduce the amount of food we eat, our bodies will be forced to draw on their fat reserves for energy in a more timely and effective manner. When glucose, which comes from carbohydrates, is not accessible, our body converts fat into energy. This happens when glucose is not readily available. This occurs more frequently at times of severe scarcity of food. The capacity of our bodies to retain fat is virtually limitless. There are many different approaches to taking part in intermittent fasting. There is no such thing as the "ideal" fasting plan, and the one you choose should truly be dependent on what will work best for you and your lifestyle. One strategy entail abstaining from food and drinks for a predetermined day, typically 12 hours.

The average individual sleeps for seven hours each night, which can be subtracted from the total time spent fasting. It is possible to quickly achieve a daily fast, which will assist your body in burning fat in a more efficient manner if you do not eat after dinner. Someone who has the habit of snacking in the evening could find that this form of fasting is beneficial to them. Although most people use it to lose weight, intermittent fasting has benefits that go well beyond that. According to research conducted on both humans and animals, it may also help you live longer that is healthier.

Intermittent fasting can be carried out in a variety of different ways. Some approaches require abstaining from food during predetermined periods each day. Some approaches call for you to abstain from food during days of the week solely. The methods used to produce varying results. If done correctly, intermittent fasting can potentially assist your body in its internal repairs and recovery. Autophagy appears to decline with age; therefore, giving yourself a boost later in life may be beneficial. However, be aware that this might not be the most effective method for shedding extra pounds and that there is no substitute for maintaining a healthy, well-rounded diet.

Made in the USA
Middletown, DE
30 January 2023